CONGENITAL HEART DISEASE

Edited by **David C. Gaze**

Congenital Heart Disease

http://dx.doi.org/10.5772/intechopen.74138
Edited by David C. Gaze

Contributors

Pedro José Curi-Curi, Juan Calderón-Colmenero, Jorge Luis Cervantes-Salazar, Samuel Ramírez-Marroquín, Shyam Sathanandam, Neil Tailor, Ranjit Philip, Ageliki Karatza, Xenophon Sinopidis, Ali Zaidi, Ayesha Salahuddin, Alice Chan, David C. Gaze

Notice

Statements and opinions expressed in the chapters are these of the individual contributors and not necessarily those of the editors or publisher. No responsibility is accepted for the accuracy of information contained in the published chapters. The publisher assumes no responsibility for any damage or injury to persons or property arising out of the use of any materials, instructions, methods or ideas contained in the book.

First published in London, United Kingdom, 2018 by IntechOpen
IntechOpen is the global imprint of INTECHOPEN LIMITED, registered in England and Wales, registration number: 11086078, The Shard, 25th floor, 32 London Bridge Street
London, SE19SG – United Kingdom
Printed in Croatia

British Library Cataloguing-in-Publication Data
A catalogue record for this book is available from the British Library

Additional hard copies can be obtained from orders@intechopen.com

Congenital Heart Disease, Edited by David C. Gaze
p. cm.
Print ISBN 978-1-78984-816-8
Online ISBN 978-1-78984-817-5

We are IntechOpen,
the world's leading publisher of
Open Access books
Built by scientists, for scientists

3,900+
Open access books available

116,000+
International authors and editors

120M+
Downloads

Our authors are among the

151
Countries delivered to

Top 1%
most cited scientists

12.2%
Contributors from top 500 universities

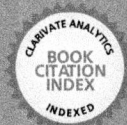

CLARIVATE ANALYTICS
BOOK CITATION INDEX
INDEXED

WEB OF SCIENCE™

Selection of our books indexed in the Book Citation Index
in Web of Science™ Core Collection (BKCI)

Interested in publishing with us?
Contact book.department@intechopen.com

Numbers displayed above are based on latest data collected.
For more information visit www.intechopen.com

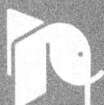

Meet the editor

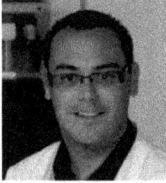

Dr. David Gaze studied biochemistry at undergraduate and Masters level in West Yorkshire followed by a PhD in Clinical Biochemistry in London, United Kingdom. He is currently Lecturer in Clinical Biochemistry at the University of Westminster and Honorary Cardiac Research Scientist within the Department of Chemical Pathology, Clinical Blood Sciences at St. George's Hospital and Medical School, London.

He has authored and co-authored in excess of 150 peer reviewed papers and 200 abstracts, as well as presented at over 50 internationally invited conferences. He has contributed five book chapters to cardiovascular related textbooks as well as writing a textbook on cardiac troponin. He is a peer reviewer for 25 medical journals. He is the commissioning editor for review articles for the *Annals of Clinical Biochemistry & Laboratory Medicine* and is Co-editor-in-chief of *Practical Laboratory Medicine*.

His academic research interests are in the development and clinical utility of cardiac biomarkers for the detection of cardiovascular disease with a special interest in the cardiorenal population.

He is a member of the Royal Society of Medicine of London; The Association for Clinical Biochemistry, of which he chairs the Clinical Sciences Review Committee for the Annals of Clinical Biochemistry. He is also a member of the American Association of Clinical Chemistry; Institute of Biomedical Sciences; Institute of Biology; European Society of Pathology; The Pathological Society of Great Britain and Ireland and associate member of the Royal Institution of London.

Gaze and colleagues have won a number of awards including two distinguished Abstract awards from the National Academy of Clinical Biochemistry as well as Diploma for Oral Presentation regarding D-dimer, natriuretic peptide and cardiac troponin in dialysis patients presented at the 17th IFCC-FESCC European Congress of Clinical Chemistry and Laboratory Medicine and the 60th National congress of the Netherlands Society of Clinical Chemistry and Laboratory Medicine in Amsterdam in 2007.

Contents

Preface

Congenital Heart Disease is a general term for a range of birth defects that affect the normal workings of the heart. It is one of the most common types of birth defect occurring in 1% of live births and affects up to 9 in every 1,000 babies born in the United Kingdom. It was estimated that 34.3 million people had a congenital heart abnormality in 2013. Abnormalities can arise in 3-5% of off spring in cases of de novo family history. Congenital heart disease was responsible for 223,000 deaths in 2010. This short volume details the common birth defects affecting the structure and functioning of the heart concentrating on the genetic basis and epidemiology, as well as risk factors, diagnostic modalities and treatment options.

Chapter 1 serves as an introduction to this short volume detailing the epidemiological prevalence of CHD over the last century. Chapter 2 examines the clinical outcomes associated with patient ductus arteriosus. Chapter 3 details the practical aspects of cardiac catheterisation interventions in patients with CHD. Chapter 4 addresses the role of ultrafiltration in patients undergoing cardiopulmonary bypass surgery for congenital abnormalities. The final chapter, chapter 5 examines the congenial abnormality coarcation of the aorta with specific reference to the adult population.

David C. Gaze
University of Westminster
London, United Kingdom

Chapter 1

Introductory Chapter: Congenital Heart Disease

David C. Gaze

Additional information is available at the end of the chapter

http://dx.doi.org/10.5772/intechopen.82217

1. Introduction

Birth defects result in abnormal physiology, often with detrimental consequences, be it physical, developmental or intellectual disability. The resulting phenotype can range from mild impairment to severe to near incompatible with life. In most extreme cases, the foetus is incompatible with life and is spontaneously aborted *prepartum*, at much distress to the parents. However, all forms are of great personal pain to the families involved.

Birth defects are broadly categorised as either structural, affecting the 'shape' of the body, or 'functional' affecting the functionality of an organ or body system, in this case, the heart and circulation. Congenital heart disease (CHD) is a non-specific medical term for a range of defects present at the time of birth that affect the normal physiology of the heart and associated circulatory system [1]. CHD can arise from a combination of genetic and environmental causes. Recent advances in molecular testing techniques aid in diagnosis of these conditions; however, this creates ethical considerations with respect to sustainability and continuity of life with such conditions, especially when treatment options to alleviate debilitating symptoms may not be available.

1.1. Epidemiology of CHD

CHD is one of the most common types of birth defects. About 28% of major congenital abnormalities are a result of a cardiac pathology [2]. These can be broadly categorised as those that result in cyanosis and those that do not (**Figure 1**). CHD occurs in approximately 1% of live births and affects up to 9 in every 1000 babies born in the United Kingdom (REF); however, the reported prevalence differs considerably globally.

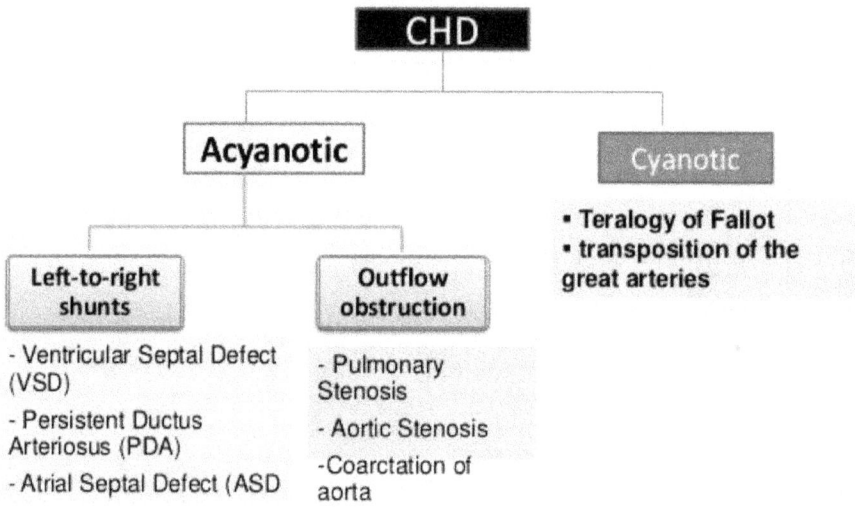

Figure 1. Broad classification of congenital heart disease.

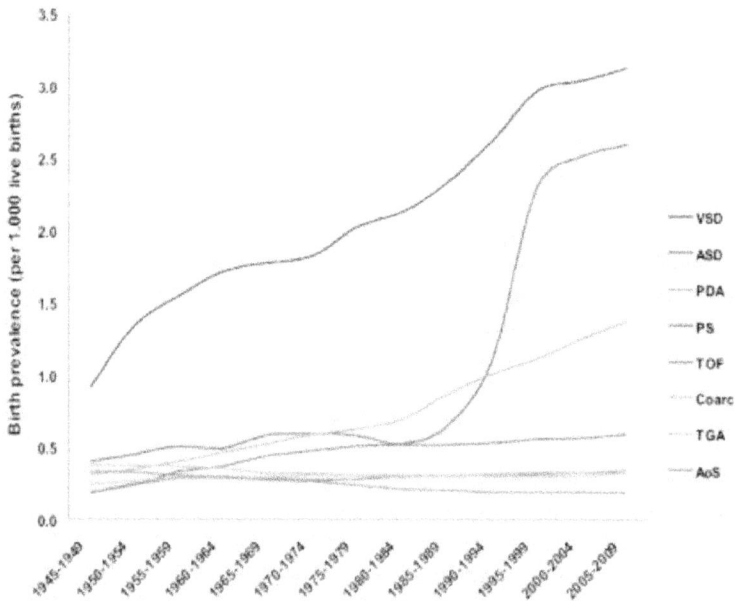

Figure 2. Prevalence of CHD between 1945 and 2009 according to defect classification. AoS, aortic stenosis; ASD, atrial septal defect; Coarc, coarctation of the aorta; PDA, patent ductus arteriosus; PS, pulmonary stenosis; TGA, transposition of the great arteries; TOF, tetralogy of Fallot; VSD, ventricular septal defect (source: [5]).

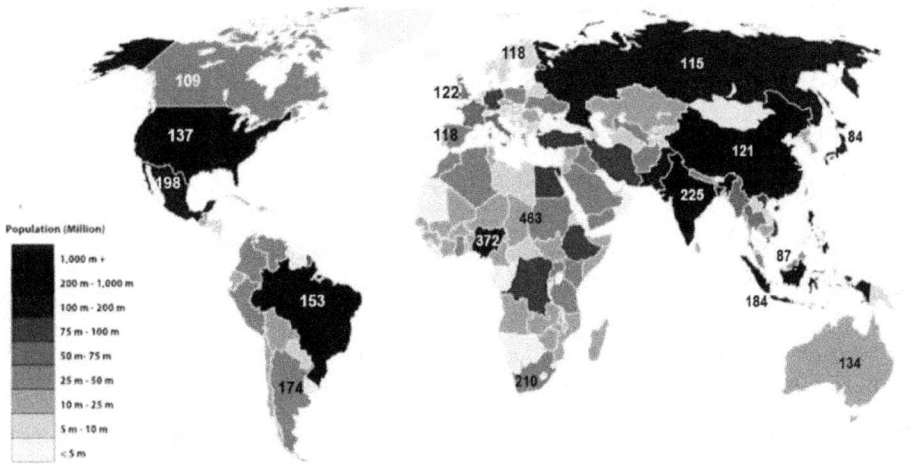

Figure 3. Global distribution of congenital heart disease in birth numbers per million population.

It was estimated that 48.9 million people had a congenital heart abnormality in 2015 [3] and CHD was responsible for 223,000 deaths in 2010 [4]. The incidence of birth defects has increased over time (**Figure 2**) partly due to the increased rates of fertility but also in part due to significant improvements in diagnostic modalities along with concomitant advances in anaesthesia and surgical intervention. The largest increase in incidence is in those born with atrial septal or ventricular septal defects.

The prevalence of CHD in the global population is illustrated in **Figure 3**. The incidence of CHD is similar between countries; however, those with higher rates of fertility have a disproportionately higher number of birth defects. Infant survival is poorest in developing countries often as a direct result of lack of medical care due to socioeconomic status. Future trends would suggest as socioeconomic conditions improve in such countries, an expected reduction in infant CHD mortality will follow.

2. Conclusion

In conclusion there is documented evidence of increasing prevalence of CHD births over the last century with a worldwide estimate of 9:1000 live births. This equates to 1.35 million annual CHD births, which has a major impact on healthcare and socioeconomic systems. The health burden falls mainly on those countries with low economic prospects, high fertility rates and poor access to advanced diagnostics and treatment options. Global healthcare monitoring and strategies to improve diagnosis and care in these areas are warranted.

Author details

David C. Gaze

Address all correspondence to: D.Gaze@westminster.ac.uk

University of Westminster, London, United Kingdom

References

[1] Mitchell SC, Korones SB, Berendes HW. Congenital heart disease in 56,109 births. Incidence and natural history. Circulation. 1971;**43**:323-332

[2] Dolk H, Loane M, Garne E, For the European Surveillance of Congenital Anomalies (EUROCAT) Working Group. Congenital heart defects in Europe: Prevalence and perinatal mortality, 2000 to 2005. Circulation. 2011;**123**:841-849

[3] GBD 2015 Disease and Injury Incidence and Prevalence. Global, regional, and national incidence, prevalence, and years lived with disability for 310 diseases and injuries, 1990-2015: A systematic analysis for the Global Burden of Disease Study 2015. Lancet. 2015;**388**:1545-1602

[4] GBD 2013 Mortality and Causes of Death, (17 December 2014). Global, regional, and national age-sex specific all-cause and cause-specific mortality for 240 causes of death, 1990-2013: A systematic analysis for the Global Burden of Disease Study 2013. Lancet. 2013;**385**:117-171

[5] Van der Linde D, Konings EEM, Slager MA, Witsenburg M, Helbing WA, Takkenberg JJM, et al. Birth prevalence of congenital heart disease world wide. A systematic review and meta-analysis. Journal of the American College of Cardiology. 2011;**58**:2241-2247

Chapter 2

Patent Arterial Duct

Ageliki A. Karatza and Xenophon Sinopidis

Additional information is available at the end of the chapter

http://dx.doi.org/10.5772/intechopen.79956

Abstract

The arterial duct is a short vessel that connects the junction of the main and left pulmonary artery to the descending aorta just distal to the left subclavian artery. In foetal life, it is an essential vascular structure that allows oxygenated blood to bypass the pulmonary circulation, since the lungs are not involved in oxygenation and enter systemic circulation. Persistent patency of the arterial duct after 3 months of age in term infants is a common form of congenital cardiovascular abnormality representing 5–10% of all congenital heart defects. Also, persistent patency of the arterial duct is a common problem in very premature sick neonates, which is associated with significant morbidity and mortality and is attributed to immaturity of the duct and associated co-morbidities in this population.

Keywords: patent arterial duct, congenital heart disease, premature neonate, ibuprofen, indomethacin, transcatheter closure, surgical ligation, Eisenmenger syndrome, foetal cardiovascular physiology, transitional circulation

1. Introduction

The arterial duct is a short vessel that derives from the distal portion of the left sixth embryonic arch and connects the junction of the main and left pulmonary artery to the descending aorta just distal to the left subclavian artery (**Figures 1–3**) [1–3]. This process is complete by the eighth week of foetal life and is necessary for normal foetal circulation and intrauterine survival [1]. During development, the arterial duct allows oxygenated blood to bypass the pulmonary circulation, since the lungs are not involved in oxygenation and enter directly into systemic circulation. After birth, the arterial duct closes via a complex biphasic process and becomes the 'ligamentum arteriosum' [4]. The arterial duct closes spontaneously in about

90% of full-term infants during the first 48 hours of life [5]. Persistent patency beyond the third month of life in term infants is a common form of congenital heart disease with an incidence of 1–2000 representing 5–10% of all congenital heart anomalies [1–3].

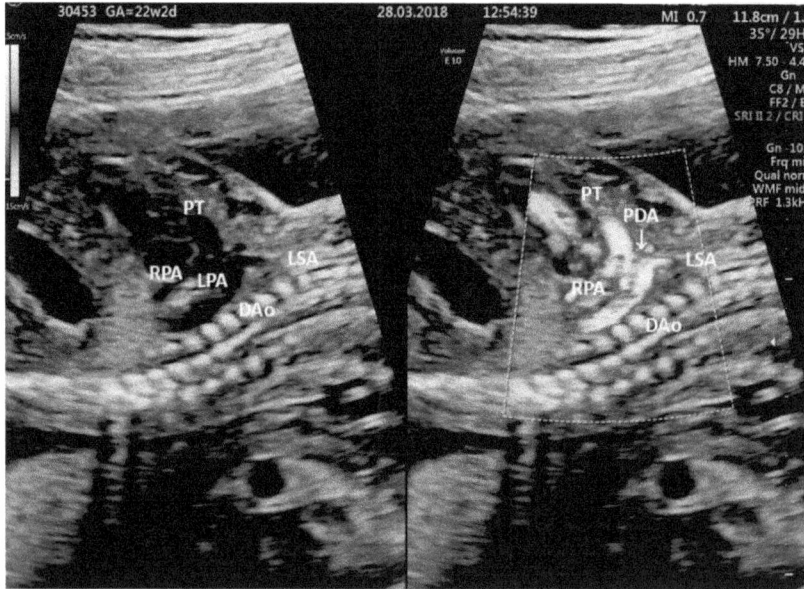

Figure 1. Saggital view of the foetal heart showing the pulmonary trunk, the aorta and the arterial duct at the same plane and the connection of the junction of the main and left pulmonary artery to the descending aorta just distal to the left subclavian artery. PT: pulmonary trunk; RPA: right pulmonary artery; LPA: left pulmonary artery; PDA: patent arterial duct; Dao: descending aorta.

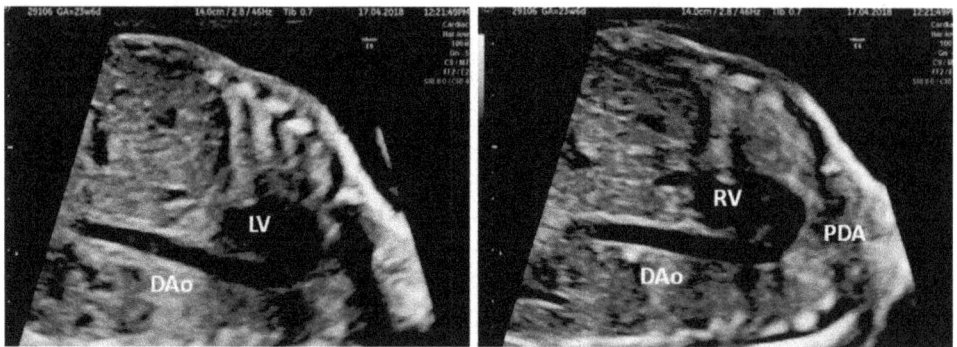

Figure 2. Saggital views of the foetal heart showing the aortic and the ductal arch. The scan angle between the ductal arch and the thoracic aorta ranges between 10° and 19° during pregnancy. Note that the ductal arch has a similar size to the aortic arch in the foetus. **Left:** *Aortic arch view.* The 'candy cane-like' aorta gives rise to the three head and neck vessels, i.e. the brachiocephalic, left common carotid and left subclavian arteries [3, 4]. **Right:** *Ductal arch view.* The arterial duct connects the main pulmonary artery to the descending aorta, forming a 'hockey stick-shaped' arch. LV: left ventricle; RV: right ventricley; PDA: patent arterial duct; Dao: descending aorta.

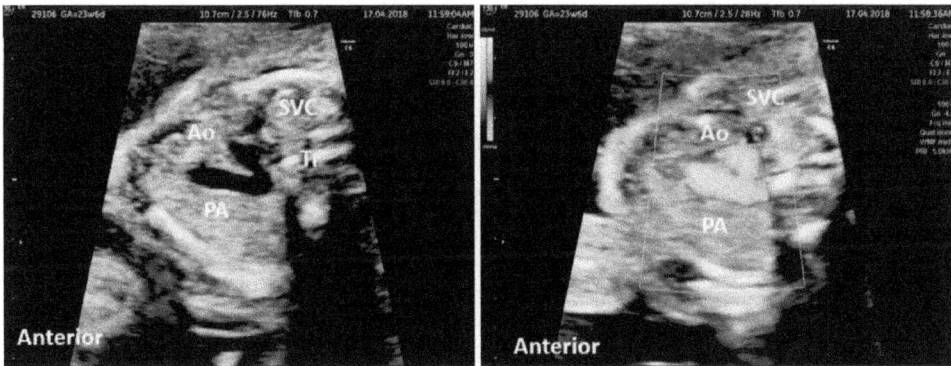

Figure 3. The '3 vessel and tracheal view' (3VT) is a standardised transverse plane of the upper mediastinum demonstrating simultaneously the course and the connection of both the aortic and ductal arches and a cross-section of the superior vena cava [1, 2]. **Left:** The three vessels are arranged in an oblique line, with the pulmonary artery in the most anterior position, the superior vena cava in the most posterior position and the aorta in between. **Right:** Transverse view of aortic and ductal arch identifies two vessels merging at the isthmus to form a V-shaped structure and Doppler imaging shows that blood flow in both arches has the same direction (blue colour). Tr: trachea; SVC: superior caval vein; Ao: aorta; PA: pulmonary artery.

Persistent patency of the arterial duct is a common problem in sick premature and extremely low-birth weight neonates, having an incidence of 65% in those weighing less than 1 kg and is associated with increased morbidity and mortality related to the consequences of a significant left-to-right shunt [6, 7].

Patent arterial duct (PAD) may present in adults with dyspnoea due to cardiac failure, pulmonary hypertension/Eisenmenger syndrome, infectious endarteritis, atrial fibrillation or be an incidental finding on routine physical examination or on transthoracic echocardiography performed for other purposes in an asymptomatic subject ('a silent duct') [8].

1.1. Normal histology and changes after birth

The arterial duct is a muscular artery and its histology is easily distinguishable from that of the aorta and pulmonary artery, the walls of which are composed of elastic fibers, which are arranged circumferentially [9]. The internal surface of the normal arterial duct is lined by a layer of endothelial cells that overlies an internal elastic lamina. The elastic lamina is fragmented and sometimes split up into several layers and is interrupted by intimal cushions that lie underneath it (**Figure 4**). The media of the ductal wall consists of two layers of smooth muscles, which have spiral arrangements in opposite directions. The outer spiral is more acute, giving the impression of circularly arranged smooth muscle fibres, whereas the inner spiral is more gradual, so the fibres appear longitudinal [9].

In utero, the patency of the arterial duct is maintained mainly due to the low oxygen tension in the foetal blood and the increased concentrations of cyclooxygenase-mediated products of arachidonic acid metabolism, primarily prostaglandin E_2 and prostacyclin [2, 10, 11]. These are produced by the duct itself and the placenta and their metabolism, which is normally performed by the pulmonary parenchyma is low, as the lungs are non-functional [2, 10, 11].

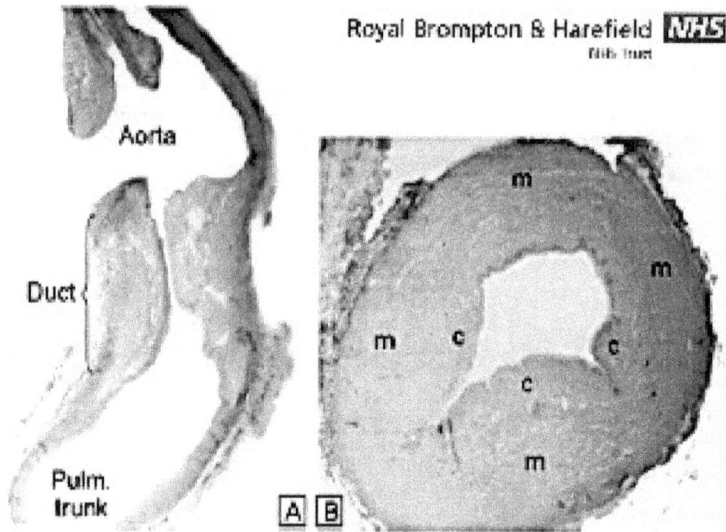

Figure 4. The 'Krichenko Classification' for anatomical classification of the PDA.

After birth, the arterial duct closes via a complex biphasic process. During the first stage, constriction of the smooth muscle in the media of the ductal wall takes place, producing shortening and thickening of the wall. These changes induce significant ischaemic hypoxia, which leads to production of several angiogenic factors and inflammatory mediators [9]. The intimal cushions disrupt the internal elastic membrane, form swollen protrusions into the ductal lumen, gradually unite and finally obliterate the lumen [9]. During the second stage of closure, proliferation of connective tissue in the intima and media takes place alongside with atrophy of smooth muscle cells and finally the arterial duct is transformed into a non-contractile ligament (the 'ligamentum arteriosum') [9].

The architecture of the arterial duct predisposes the tissue to contraction and lumen obliteration under appropriate signals and conditions, such as the increase in oxygen tension that normally takes place after birth [15]. Furthermore, there are various vasoactive substances such as bradykinin and endogenous catecholamines, which also mediate ductal closure after birth [9]. Prostaglandins exert an effect on ductal wall that is opposite to oxygen, causing relaxation of the smooth muscles, and inhibit the obliteration of the lumen [9]. However, their concentrations normally decrease after birth due to the removal of the placenta and their metabolism by the lungs [2].

1.2. Epidemiology and aetiology

In normal term infants, the closure of the arterial duct may be delayed until 3 months of life, after which the incidence of spontaneous closure is very low [1, 3]. If the duct remains open beyond 3 months of life in full-term infants, it is termed 'persistently patent arterial duct' and its patency has been attributed to inherent abnormality of the ductal tissue and/or signalling pathways that normally trigger its closure [12]. However, the exact mechanisms as to why the duct will not close in some full-term infants remain unknown [3].

Also, the incidence of PAD in infants and children born at full term is not precisely known due to the fact that most subjects are asymptomatic. Before the widespread use of echocardiography, the incidence of clinically evident persistent PAD was reported to be about 1 in 2000 births, which accounts for approximately 5–10% of all congenital heart defects [1–3]. If cases detected incidentally by echocardiography are included, the incidence will be much higher and is estimated to be 1:500 [1, 3].

The female-to-male ratio for PDA is about 2:1. In addition, PAD occurs with increased frequency in several genetic syndromes, including Down syndrome (trisomy 21), trisomy 18, Char syndrome (autosomal dominant), Carpenter syndrome (single gene mutation), Holt-Oram syndrome (autosomal dominant) and incontinentia pigmenti (X-linked). Although, most cases are sporadic, there is increasing evidence that genetic factors are involved in many patients. Prenatal infection, such as rubella, may also play a role in some cases [1, 3].

1.3. Anatomy and histology

A universally accepted system for anatomical classification of the PAD is the 'Krichenko Classification', which is based on the angiographic appearance of the duct [14]. The five Krichenko PDA subtypes are: type A (conical), type B (window type), type C (tubular), type D (complex) and type E (elongated), with a relative incidence of approximately 85% for type A, 10% for both types D and E combined and 5% for both types B and C combined [13] (**Figure 5**). Most commonly, a patent arterial duct occurs as an isolated congenital heart defect. Histologically, the internal elastic lamina of the PAD is generally intact and the intimal cushions are absent or are less well formed than normal [14] (**Figure 6**). Morphologically, a progressive transformation of the duct wall to the elastic-type artery has been observed with light microscopy. In this transformation, three stages were determined—stage I: laminar elastosis of the intima; stage II: same as stage I plus incomplete elastic transformation of the media and stage III: fully developed elastic-type artery [14].

However, in normal subjects, selective constriction of arterial duct suggests the presence of highly specialised contractile mechanisms. Indeed, smooth muscles in arterial duct are more differentiated compared to those in other arteries, which may be one of the cellular mechanisms responsible for the closure of the arterial duct after birth [15].Postnatal constriction

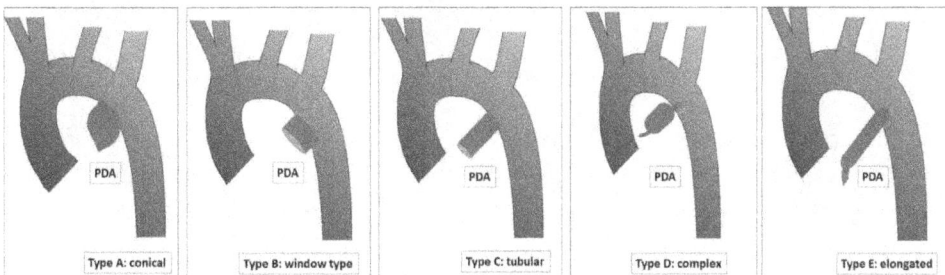

| Type A: conical | Type B: window type | Type C: tubular | Type D: complex | Type E: elongated |

Figure 5. Histologic sections through two normal ducts from neonates. (a)This longitudinal section shows the distinctive appearance of the ductal wall composed mainly of smooth muscle compared to the walls of the aorta and pulmonary trunk, which are composed primarily of elastic tissue. (b) This transverse section shows the intimal cushions (c) that protrude towards the ductal lumen. m = media. [trichrome stain].

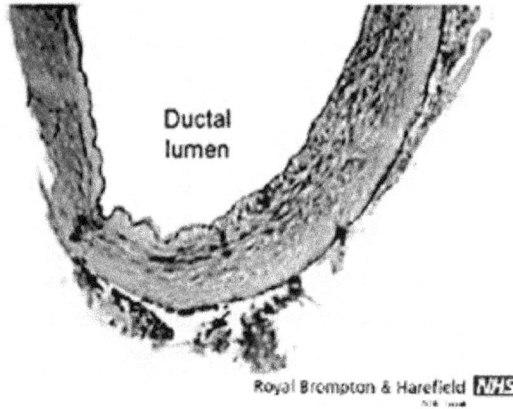

Ductal
lumen

Royal Brompton & Harefield [NHS]

Figure 6. Histology image showing part of a persistently patent duct cut in cross-section. The internal elastic lamina is intact and appears as a black line lining the ductal lumen. Intimal cushions are barely formed, leaving a widely patent lumen. [elastic van Geison stain].

of the full-term arterial duct arteriosus produces cell death and remodelling of its wall. The extensive degree of cell death that occurs in the newborn duct after birth is associated primarily with ATP depletion. The increased glycolytic capacity of the immature duct may enable it to tolerate episodes of hypoxia and nutrient shortage, making it more resistant to developing postnatal cell death and permanent obliteration of its lumen [16].

1.4. Pathophysiology and clinical picture

After birth, systemic resistance increases markedly as the placenta is disconnected from the systemic circulation, and pulmonary vascular resistance decreases significantly over time [10, 11, 17]. Therefore, in patients in which the arterial duct remains persistently patent, the direction of flow is left-to-right and the amount of shunt is determined by the difference in systemic and pulmonary vascular resistance, as well as by the resistance to blood flow determined by the residual diameter, geometry and distensibility of the duct (**Figures 7–9**) [18].

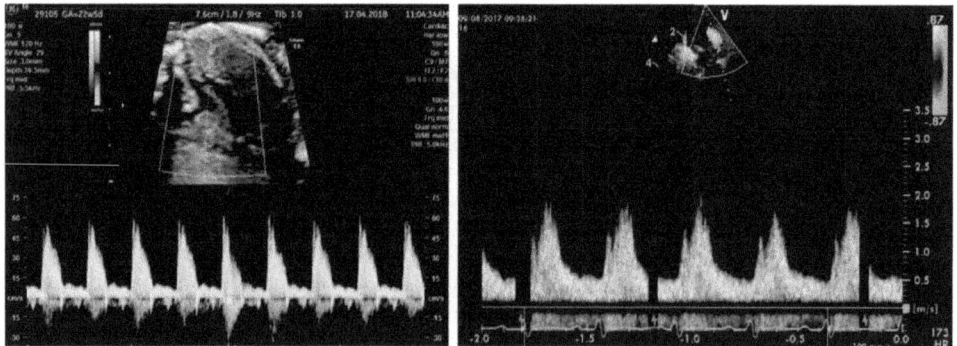

Figure 7. Left: Normal (right-to-left) ductal Doppler in a 22-week + 5–day-old foetus. **Right:** Left-to-right ductal Doppler in an extremely premature neonate showing a similar pulsatile unrestrictive, but reversed, pattern of flow.

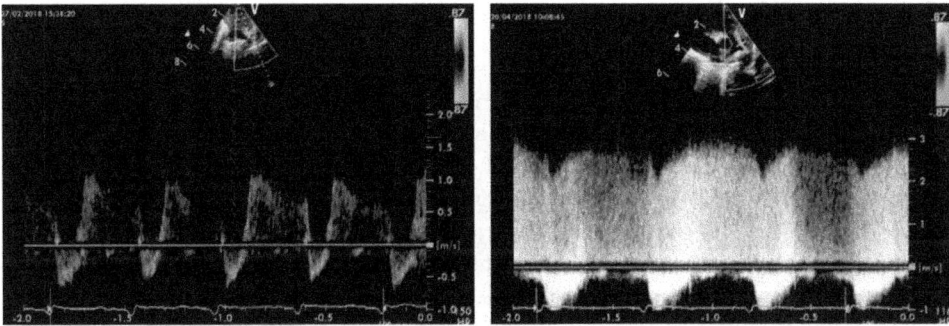

Figure 8. Left: Early postnatal ductal Doppler, which is bi-directional with predominant left-to right, suggesting a decline of pulmonary resistance after birth. **Right:** Late postnatal restrictive ductal Doppler, which is pure left-to right, suggesting further decline of pulmonary resistance and a normal adaptation to extra-uterine life.

In patients with isolated persistency of the arterial duct, the clinical manifestations and complications are mainly related to the degree of pulmonary over-circulation and left ventricular volume overload [1–3, 12]. The increased pulmonary venous return to the left heart results in increased left ventricular volume and end-diastolic pressure, as well as increased left atrial size and pressure. The left ventricle compensates by increasing stroke volume, and eventually may hypertrophy in order to normalise wall stress [1].

Most patients are asymptomatic when the duct is small. In a moderate-to-large duct, infants may have increased work of breathing, which becomes manifest as fast or laboured breathing and tiredness during feeds. In older children, there may be a history of exertional dyspnoea. Large shunts may lead to failure to thrive, recurrent respiratory tract infections and congestive heart failure [1, 2]. In patients with long-standing moderate-to-large left-to-right shunt, irreversible pulmonary vascular changes may occur over time, secondary to prolonged exposure to high pulmonary blood flow [3, 12]. These changes include arteriolar medial hypertrophy, intimal proliferation and fibrosis. When pulmonary arterial pressure exceeds systemic pressure, the flow across the duct is reversed and right-to-left shunting occurs (Eisenmenger syndrome) [18].

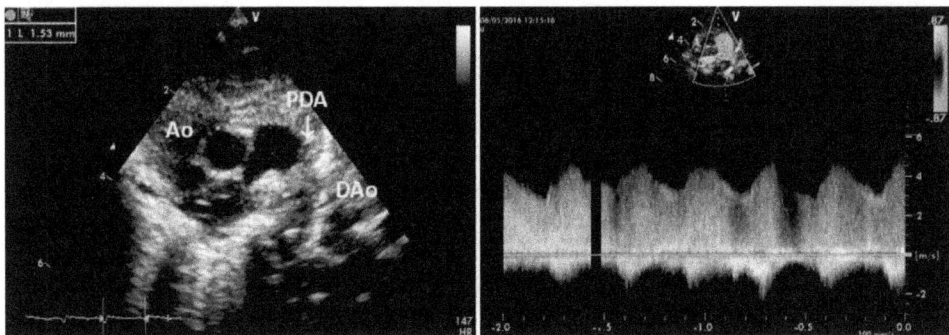

Figure 9. Left: 'ductal shot' which is a modified shot axis view showing a patent arterial duct measuring 1.53 mm (the 'three leg stool appearance'). **Right:** Non-restrictive ductal Doppler in the same patient. Ao: aorta; PDA: patent arterial duct; Dao: descending aorta. Ao: aorta; PT: pulmpnary trunk; Dao: descending aorta; PDA device: Amplatzer duct occluder.

1.5. Physical examination

Physical examination findings depend on the size of the patent arterial duct and the presence of associated defects. A small PAD presents with a continuous 'machinery' type murmur, which is best heard at the left infraclavicular area [1–3, 12]. In case of a large duct with pure left-to-right shunt, besides the classic 'machinery' murmur, there may be bounding peripheral pulses due to hyperdynamic circulation and a wide pulse pressure. Adults with a large, non-restrictive PDA, however, may have suprasystemic pulmonary artery pressure and develop Eisenmenger physiology with a right-to-left shunt. In these patients, the continuous 'machinery' murmur is no longer audible. They may develop differential cyanosis, with more profound desaturation of the lower extremities associated with clubbing, which is more prominent in the toes. This represents the most specific physical sign of a large PAD associated with shunt reversal [20]. On the contrary, a trivial arterial duct is totally asymptomatic, flow through it is minimal and non-turbulent and thus no murmur is audible [1–3].

1.6. Specific age groups

1.6.1. Patent arterial duct in the preterm neonate

Prematurity increases the likelihood of persistent ductal patency, which is seen in about 30% of very low-birth weight and up to 65% of extremely low-birth weight infants [21]. The incidence of patent arterial duct increases with decreasing gestational age. The inherent immaturity in the muscular wall of the duct in preterm infants is associated with decreased oxygen sensitivity and increased sensitivity to prostaglandins and nitric oxide, leading to reduced ductal constriction. Without sufficient enough physiologic hypoxia to promote vascular remodelling, anatomic closure will not occur and the duct may fail to close or reopen after closure [21]. Also, very premature infants usually have respiratory distress syndrome and relatively low oxygen levels after birth, contributing to delayed effective ductal closure [10, 22]. Although the duct, the preterm newborn continues to respond to PGE2 after birth, it becomes less dependent on prostaglandins and more dependent on other vasodilators during the weeks following delivery. This could explain why the effectiveness of prostaglandin inhibitors, as a pharmacologic treatment to promote ductal closure, wanes with increasing postnatal age [23].

The pathophysiologic features of a PAD depend both on the magnitude of the left-to-right shunt and on the cardiac and pulmonary responses to the shunt. The consequences may include pulmonary over-circulation and/or systemic hypoperfusion [24]. Despite the ability of the left ventricle to increase its output in the setting of a significant left-to-right shunt, 'ductal steal' occurs, resulting in hypoperfusion of peripheral organs (**Figures 10 and 11**). Also, the decreased ability of the preterm infant to maintain active pulmonary vasoconstriction combined by the use of surfactant replacement therapy in preterm infants with respiratory distress syndrome lead to a more rapid drop in pulmonary vascular resistance and exacerbate the magnitude of left-to-right shunt. This results in lung congestion and volume overload of the preterm left atrium and ventricle (**Figure 12**) [22]. Although 75% of premature infants with PAD at discharge from the neonatal intensive care unit will have spontaneous closure during the first year of life, prolonged exposure to PAD has been associated with significant morbidity, and a four to sevenfold increase in mortality [21]. Complications associated with a

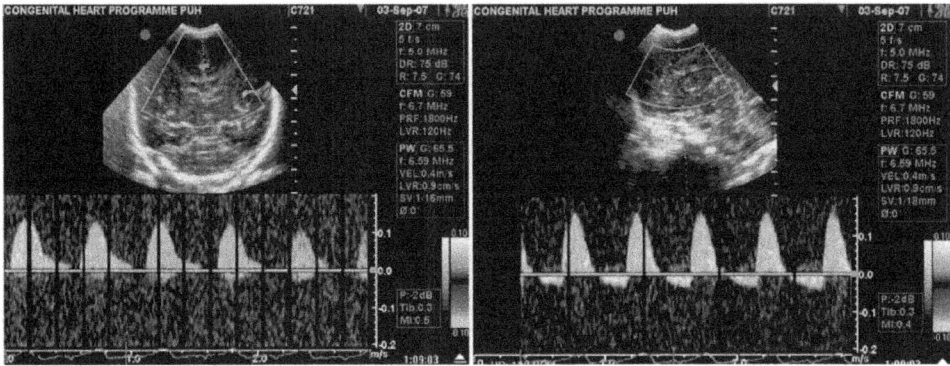

Figure 10. Abnormal middle cerebral artery Doppler with absence of end-diastolic flow (left) and reversal of end-diastolic flow (right) predisposing to intra/periventricular haemorrhage.

patent arterial duct in preterm infants include peri/intraventricular haemorrhage, necrotising enterocolitis, renal failure, congestive heart failure with hypotension and metabolic acidosis, haemorrhagic pulmonary oedema and prolonged ventilator dependence with subsequent chronic lung disease [21].

Whether to treat or not, as well as when to treat a PAD, has been a controversial topic for the past decade [21, 24, 25]. It has become apparent from systematic review of the literature that there is no clear evidence of effect on long-term outcomes of treating PAD, which some authors consider a physiologic phenomenon in sick preterm infants [23, 24].

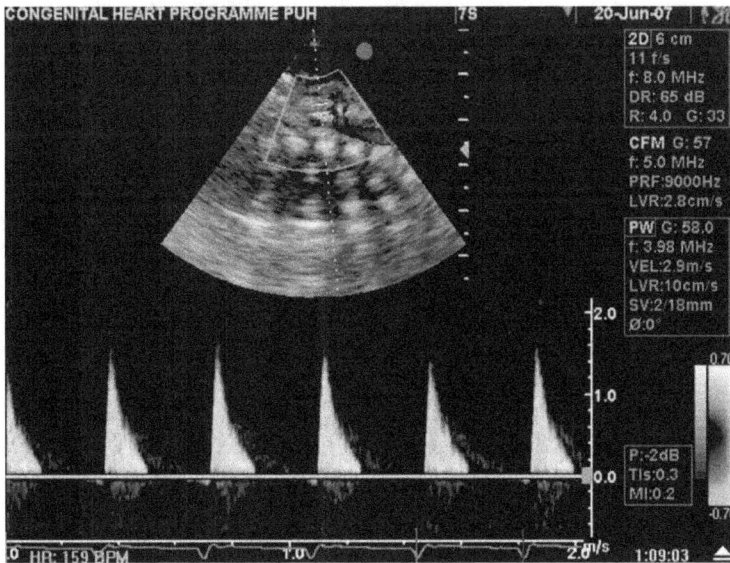

Figure 11. Abnormal superior mesenteric artery Doppler with absence of end-diastolic flow predisposing to necrotising enterocolitis.

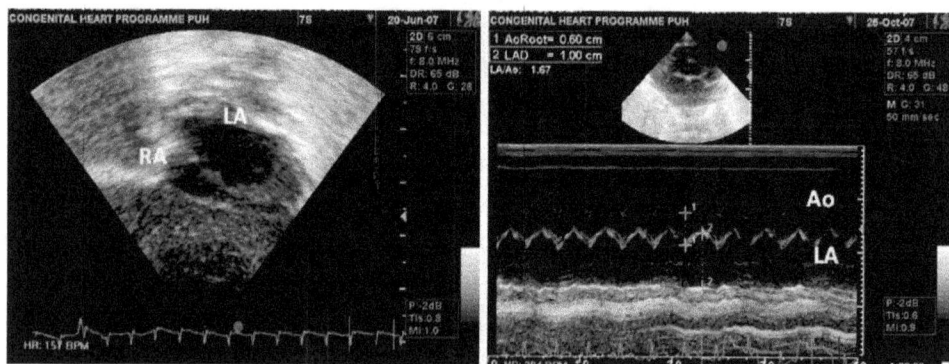

Figure 12. Left atrial dilatation (left) as a result of a significant left-to-right shunt with left atrium in systole to aorta in diastole ratio (right), LA/Ao = 1.67 (normal values<1.40). RA: right atrium; LA: left atrium; Ao: aorta.

Non-steroidal anti-inflammatory drugs have been traditionally used to close PADs to prevent associated complications [21, 24]. As a large proportion of the PADs in preterm infants will spontaneously close within the first few days, in recent years emphasis has been given to targeted treatment of PADs when considered haemodynamically significant based on clinical and echocardiographic criteria. The two most commonly used treatment options are intravenous ibuprofen and intravenous indomethacin [21, 24]. Recent observational studies suggest that paracetamol may have a role in PAD closure in infants who are resistant to conventional treatment or those with contraindications to conventional medical therapy [26]. A recent meta-analysis which included preterm infants treated with intravenous or oral indomethacin, ibuprofen, acetaminophen, placebo or no treatment concluded that high doses of oral ibuprofen are associated with a higher likelihood of closure of a haemodynamically significant PAD versus standard doses of intravenous ibuprofen or intravenous indomethacin. However, placebo or no treatment did not significantly change the risk of mortality, necrotising enterocolitis or intraventricular haemorrhage [27].

1.6.2. Adults with untreated patent arterial duct

The mortality in adults with an unoperated PAD is estimated to be 1–1.5% in the third decade, 2–2.5% in the fourth decade and increases by 4% per year thereafter, with 33% mortality at the age of 40 and 60% at 60 years of life [28]. Untreated PAD may cause congestive heart failure due to left heart volume overload and increased pulmonary blood flow; atrial fibrillation or flutter due to atrial enlargement; infective endocarditis/endarteritis, which is more common in the second or third decade of life; lower respiratory tract infections; calcification and pulmonary vascular disease/Eisenmenger syndrome [20]. Adult patients with Eisenmenger syndrome have dyspnoea on exertion, fatigue, syncope due to low systemic cardiac output, neurologic abnormalities due to secondary erythrocytosis and hyperviscosity, right heart failure, arrhythmias and haemoptysis due to pulmonary infarction [19].

Other more uncommon complications include aneurysmal dilatation of the duct, recurrent laryngeal nerve paralysis due to compression from a dilated pulmonary artery, peripheral emboli and exceedingly rarely aortic or pulmonary artery dissection [19, 20, 29].

Echocardiography is the key diagnostic imaging modality; however, it may be difficult in patients with Eisenmenger physiology [30]. Echocardiography defines the presence and the size of the PAD, the effect of the shunt on the left atrium and left ventricle, the pulmonary circulation and any associated lesions [31]. Magnetic resonance imaging (MRI) or computed tomography (CT) is indicated to evaluate pulmonary artery anatomy or to obtain more precise left ventricular volumes. Cardiac catheterisation is reserved for cases with signs of pulmonary hypertension on echocardiography to estimate pulmonary vascular resistance and assess the reactivity of the pulmonary vascular bed [30, 31].

Transcatheter occlusion is the treatment of choice, even if operation for associated anomalies has been scheduled. In adults, the duct is often calcified and the tissue in the area of the aortic isthmus and pulmonary artery is friable, making surgical ligation difficult and more hazardous compared to paediatric patients [30, 31]. Surgical ligation is thus reserved for patients with very large ducts, those with difficult anatomy or aneurysmal dilatation [30].

Arterial duct occlusion eliminates volume overload of the left ventricle and pulmonary over-circulation, treats congestive heart failure and prevents both the development of obstructive pulmonary vascular disease/Eisenmenger syndrome and subacute endocarditis/endarteritis [1–3, 29]. Routine follow-up is recommended every 3–5 years for patients with a small PAD without evidence of left-heart volume overload. Also, follow-up approximately every 5 years for patients who received a device is recommended because of the lack of long-term data [20].

2. Management: surgical and transcatheter techniques

Over the past 15–20 years, transcatheter closure of PADs has become the standard of care for most patients and surgery is reserved for those with very large ducts or low-weight babies (**Figures 13** and **14**) [6]. A number of studies have been published reporting experience with transcatheter PAD closure, in particular using detachable coils and the Amplatzer ductal occluder device [6, 29]. In the reported series of transcatheter closure, major procedural events occurred in 1.0% of cases, a risk not related to ductal size [6]. The procedural risks specifically associated with closure of a silent duct are not known.

According to the scientific statement from the American Heart Association (AHA) concerning cardiac catheterisation and intervention in paediatric cardiac disease, transcatheter PAD closure is indicated for the treatment of a moderate-sized or large PAD with left-to-right shunt associated with congestive heart failure, failure to thrive, an enlarged left atrium or left ventricle or pulmonary over-circulation, provided the anatomy and patient size are suitable (**Figure 15**) [29].

Transcatheter PAD occlusion is considered reasonable in the presence of a small left-to-right shunt with normal-sized heart chambers when the PAD is audible by standard auscultation techniques [29]. Small PADs without haemodynamic overload are generally closed because of the risk of subacute bacterial endocarditis [29, 32].

In the current era, transcatheter techniques are used to close PADs in most patients who weigh more than 5–6 kg [33]. The size and stiffness of the delivery sheath limit this approach in infants with low body weight; however, transcatheter occlusion has been applied with good success in symptomatic infants as small as 1800 g to avoid thoracotomy and the complications

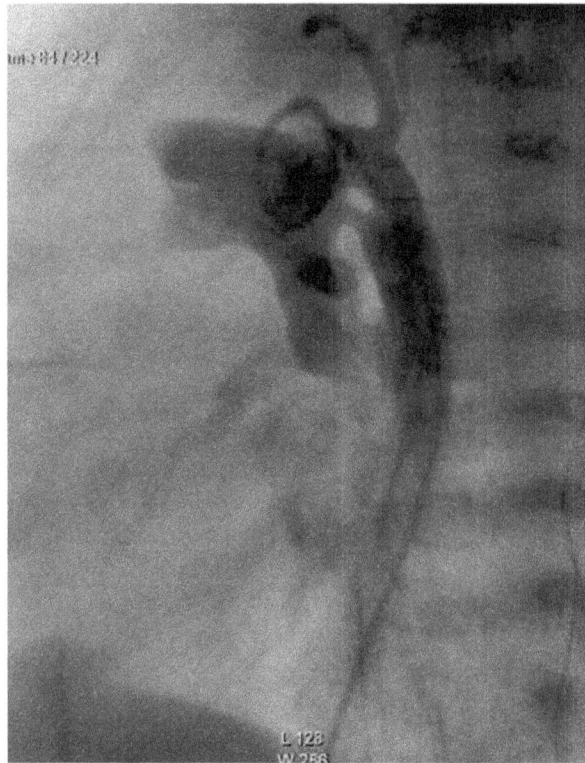

Figure 13. Angiography prior to transcatheter closure attempt showing a large patent arterial duct.

associated with surgical ligation [34]. Excellent results have been achieved using coil devices or plugs implanted into the arterial duct via the descending thoracic aorta using a transfemoral approach. Potential complications include device embolization, vascular injury, partial occlusion of the left pulmonary artery or aorta by the plug, and residual shunting [33]. Surgical strategies are applied for the larger arterial duct. The most typical surgical management of a PAD in older children is with ligation and division of the duct through a left thoracotomy.

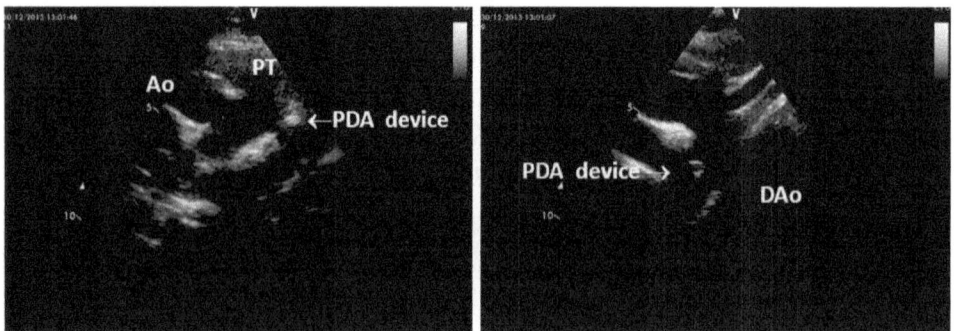

Figure 14. Patient of **Figure 9** after successful amplatzer duct occlusion showing the device in correct position. **Left:** aortic arch view. **Right:** short axis view.

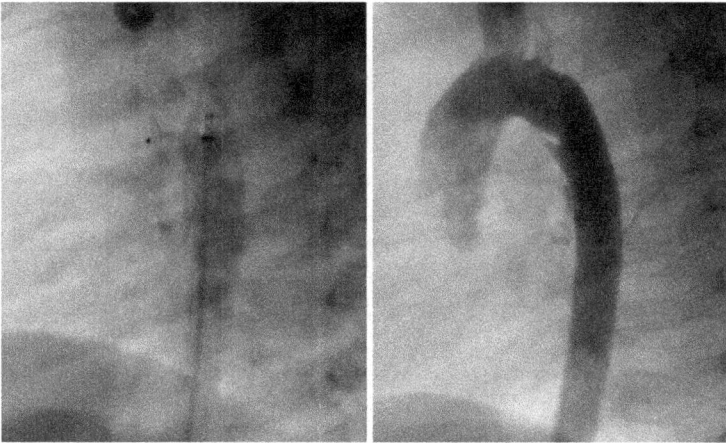

Figure 15. Left: Angiography during transcatheter closure attempt with an Amplatzer duct occluder. Right: angiography showing successful PAD closure in the same patient.

Video-assisted thoracoscopic PAD ligation is a less invasive technique that may be considered for selected patients [35]. Unsuccessfully performed thoracoscopic surgeries can safely be converted to conventional thoracotomy. Video-assisted thoracoscopic surgery is a less invasive approach, leads to a better aesthetic effect and lower surgical complication rate [35]. The postoperative management of older infants and children is usually quite straightforward. Most patients have a substantial improvement in the haemodynamic efficiency of the heart following this operation and do not require inotropic support or significant manipulation of the systemic and pulmonary vasculature in the perioperative period [33].

In premature babies and small infants, simple double ligation is performed. Surgical PAD closure may be considered for patients who do not respond to medical management, or if medical management is contraindicated [33]. A subset of premature neonates develop transient haemodynamic instability characterised by left ventricular dysfunction, low cardiac output syndrome and the need for increased respiratory support. Patients weighing less than 1000 g are at particular risk, likely related to the immaturity of the myocardium [33]. Although uncommon, a number of complications may develop following surgical PAD ligation. Residual shunting may uncommonly occur through a PAD that has been ligated but not divided. Because the recurrent laryngeal nerve travels around the PAD, consideration should be given to prevent potential injury to the nerve during duct ligation [33].

3. Current controversies

3.1. Infective endocarditis/endarteritis prophylaxis

Subacute bacterial endocarditis/endarteritis has been reported in both symptomatic and asymptomatic patients with a patent arterial duct; however, the necessity for subacute endocarditis prophylaxis remains to be defined [36–38]. Infective endocarditis is an uncommon but life-threatening disease and prevention is preferable to treatment of established infection.

Bacteraemia with organisms known to cause infective endocarditis occurs commonly in association with invasive dental, gastrointestinal or genitourinary tract procedures. However, infective endocarditis is much more likely to result from frequent exposure to random bacteraemias associated with daily activities. Although prophylaxis may prevent an exceedingly small number of cases of infective endocarditis in individuals who undergo a dental, gastrointestinal tract or genitourinary tract procedure, the risk of antibiotic-associated adverse events exceeds the benefit. Therefore, maintenance of optimal oral health and hygiene may reduce the incidence of bacteraemia from daily activities and is more important than prophylactic antibiotics for a dental procedure to reduce the risk of infective endocarditis. These were the primary reasons for the revision of the infective endocarditis prophylaxis guidelines of the American Heart Association Committee on Rheumatic Fever, Endocarditis and Kawasaki disease, which does not recommend routine subacute bacterial endocarditis prophylaxis for unrepaired PAD [32].

The impacts of the application of the 2007 AHA antibiotic prophylaxis guidelines for infective endocarditis were studied using a nationally representative cohort of paediatric patients in the US. The data did not demonstrate significant changes on the overall incidence or severity of paediatric infective endocarditis in the period 2001–2012 [37]. However, a significant increase in disease incidence trend due to viridans group streptococci was observed in the 10–17 age group in the postguideline period. Infective endocarditis due to viridans group streptococci is presumed to result principally from bacteraemia during dental work, which is more common in older children. It should be noted that the absence of overall change in infective endocarditis incidence from pre- to postguideline might in part reflect poor adherence to the 2007 AHA policy [39, 40].

3.2. The 'silent arterial duct'

With the advent of novel ultrasound technologies, the incidence of persistent patency of the arterial duct is expected to become much higher. If cases detected incidentally on transthoracic echocardiography performed for other purposes are included, the incidence is estimated to be 1:500 individuals [1–3, 20]. When the duct becomes very small, flow is diminished and non-turbulent and thus no murmur is audible. The very small duct, which is identified incidentally in asymptomatic subjects and produces no murmur on auscultation, is termed 'the silent arterial duct' [10, 29].

There is still controversy related to the need of closure of a silent arterial duct which is associated with a small left-to-right shunt, a normal heart size and an inaudible murmur (AHA Class of recommendation IIb; Level of evidence C) [29]. There are few data supporting significant benefits of occluding it solely to prevent subacute infective endocarditis. A tiny patent arterial duct does not have a high enough velocity of flow through it to cause endothelial damage, which is the substrate for bacterial growth [20]. According to the European Society of Cardiology (ESC), device closure should be considered in small PADs with continuous murmur, normal left ventricular and pulmonary artery pressure (Level of Evidence IIa; Class of Recommendation C C), but should be avoided in the silent duct (Level of Evidence III; Class of Reccommendation C) [29].

4. Conclusion

A patent arterial duct is a cardiovascular disorder documented in patients of all ages, from extremely premature infants to elderly subjects [41, 42]. Currently, the widespread availability of echocardiography has resulted in improved detection and detailed characterisation of the size of a PAD, the effects on the left atrium and left ventricle, the pulmonary circulation and any associated lesions. The haemodynamic consequences of PDA are analogous to the magnitude and the direction of the shunt, which depends on the flow resistance within the duct, and the dynamic pressure gradient between the pulmonary and systemic blood flow [42]. Catheter occlusion is the treatment of choice and surgical ligation is reserved for patients with very large ducts or when interventional closure is not feasible. However, the optimal management of the 'silent arterial duct' remains controversial and requires further investigation.

Acknowledgements

The authors would like to thank professor Vassileios Papadopoulos and Dr. Konstantinos Tziveriotis, Academic Obstetricians of the feto-maternal Unit at the University of Patras Medical School for the provision of the foetal images.

Conflict of interest

The authors declare that there are no real or potential conflicts of interest.

A. Appendix 1

[1] The application of classification of recommendations and level of evidence according to AHA/ACC is published in *Circulation* [43].

[2] The recommendations for formulating and issuing ESC Guidelines can be found on the ESC Web Site. (http://www.escardio.org/ guidelines-surveys/esc-guidelines/about/Pages/rules writing.aspx).

B. Appendix 2

Further reading regarding assessment of a PAD with foetal and neonatal echocardiography. See Ref. [43].

Author details

Ageliki A. Karatza[1]* and Xenophon Sinopidis[2]

*Address all correspondence to: agelikikaratza@hotmail.com

1 Department of Paediatrics, University of Patras Medical School, Patras, Greece

2 Department of Paediatric Surgery, University of Patras Medical School, Patras, Greece

References

[1]   Schneider DJ. The patent ductus arteriosus in term infants, children and adults. Seminars in Perinatology. 2012;**36**(2):146-153

[2]   Schneider DJ, Moore JW. Patent ductus arteriosus. Circulation. 2006;**114**(917):1873-1882

[3]   Anilkumar M. Patent ductus arteriosus. Cardiology Clinics. 2013;**31**(3):417-430

[4]   Huff T, Bhimji SS. Anatomy, Thorax, Heart, Ductus Arteriosus. StatPearls [Internet]. Treasure Island (FL): StatPearls Publishing; 2018-2017

[5]   Kang C, Zhao E, Zhou Y, Zhao H, Liu Y, Gao N, et al. Dynamic changes of pulmonary arterial pressure and ductus arteriosus in human newborns from birth to 72 hours of age. Medicine (Baltimore). 2016;**95**(3):e2599

[6]   Baruteau AE, Hascoët S, Baruteau J, Boudjemline Y, Lambert V, Angel CY, et al. Trans-catheter closure of patent ductus arteriosus. Past, present and future. Archives of Cardio-vascular Diseases. 2014;**107**(2):122-132

[7]   Garcia AV, Luckish J. Minimally invasive patent ductus arteriosus ligation. Clinics in Perinatology. 2017;**44**(4):763-771

[8]   Fortescue EB, Lock JE, Galvin T, McElhinney DB. To close or not to close: The very small patent ductus arteriosus. Congenital Heart Disease. 2010;**5**(4):354-365

[9]   Marsui H, McCarthy KP, Ho SY. Morphology of the patent arterial duct: Features relevant to treatment. Images in Paediatric Cardiology. 2008;**10**(1):27-38

[10] Finnemore A, Groves A. Physiology of the fetal and transitional circulation. Seminars in Fetal & Neonatal Medicine. 2015;**20**(4):210-216

[11] Morton S. Fetal physiology and the transition to extrauterine life. Clinics in Perinatology. 2016;**43**(3):395-407

[12] Forsey JT, Elmasry OA, Martin RP. Patent arterial duct. Orphanet Journal of Rare Diseases. 2009;**4**:17

[13] Ho SY, Anderson RH. Anatomical closure of the ductus arteriosus: A study in 35 specimens. Journal of Anatomy. 1979;**128**(4):829-836

[14] Chuaqui B, Piwonka G, Farrú O. The wall in persistent ductus arteriosus (Author's translation). (article in German). Virchows Archiv. A, Pathological Anatomy and Histology. 1977;**372**(4):315-324

[15] Kim HS, Aikawa M, Kimura K, Kuro-o M, Nakahara K, Suzuki T, et al. Ductus arteriosus. Advanced differentiation of smooth muscle cells demonstrated by myosin heavy chain isoform expression in rabbits. Circulation, 1810. 1993;**88**(4 Pt 1):1804

[16] Levin M, Goldbarg S, Lindqvist A, Swärd K, Roman C, Liu BM, et al. ATP depletion and cell death in the neonatal lamb ductus arteriosus. Pediatric Research. 2005;**57**(6):801-805

[17] Evans NJ, Archer LN. Postnatal circulatory adaptation in healthy term and preterm neonates. Archives of Disease in Childhood. 1990;**65**(10):24-26

[18] Tomita H, Fuse S, Hatakeyama K, Chiba S. Epinephrine-induced constriction of the persistent ductus arteriosus and its relation to distensibility. Japanese Circulation Journal. 1998;**62**(12):913-914

[19] Mebus S, Schulze-Neick I, Oechslin E, Niwa K, Trindade PT, Hager A, Hess J, Kaemmerer H. The adult patient with Eisenmenger syndrome: A medical update after Dana Point Part I: Epidemiology, clinical aspects and diagnostic options. Current Cardiology Reviews. 2010; **6**(4):356-362

[20] Warnes CA, Williams RG, Bashore TM, Child JS, Connolly HM, Dearani JA, et al. ACC/ AHA 2008 Guidelines for the Management of Adults With Congenital Heart Disease. A report of the American College of Cardiology/American Heart Association Task Force on Practice Guidelines (Writing Committee to Develop Guidelines on the Management of Adults With Congenital Heart Disease). Circulation. 2008;**118**(23):e714-e833

[21] Prescott S, Keim-Malpass J. Patent ductus arteriosus in the preterm infant. diagnostic and treatment options. Advances in Neonatal Care. 2017;**17**(1):10-18

[22] Evans N. Preterm patent ductus arteriosus: A continuing conundrum for the neonatologist? Seminars in Fetal & Neonatal Medicine. 2015;**20**(4):272-277

[23] Teixeira LS, McNamara PJ. Enhanced intensive care for the neonatal ductus arteriosus. Acta Paediatrica. 2006;**95**(4):394-403

[24] EL-Khuffash A, Weisz DA, PJ MN. Reflections of the changes in patent ductus arteriosus management during the last 10 years. Archives of Disease in Childhood. Fetal and Neonatal Edition. 2016;**101**(5):F474-F478

[25] Mitra S, Rønnestad A, Holmstrøm H. Management of patent ductus arteriosus in preterm infants—Where do we stand? Congenital Heart Disease. 2013;**8**(6):500-512

[26] Hammerman C, Bin-Nun A, Markovitch E, Schimmel MS, Kaplan M, Fink D. Ductal closure with paracetamol: A surprising new approach to patent ductus arteriosus treatment. Pediatrics. 2011;**128**(6):e1618-e1621

[27] Mitra S, Florez ID, Tamayo ME, Mbuagbaw L, Vanniyasingam T, Veroniki AA, et al. Association of placebo, indomethacin, ibuprofen, and acetaminophen with closure of

hemodynamically significant patent ductus arteriosus in preterm infants: A systematic review and meta-analysis. Journal of the American Medical Association. 2018;**319**(12): 1221-1238

[28] Campbell M. Natural history of persistent ductus arteriosus. British Heart Journal. 1968; **30**(1):4-13

[29] Feltes TF, Bacha E, Beekman RH 3rd, Cheatham JP, Feinstein JA, Gomes AS, et al. Indications for cardiac catheterization and intervention in pediatric cardiac disease: A scientific statement from the American Heart Association. Circulation. 2011;**123**(22):2607-2652

[30] Chugh R, Salem MM. Echocardiography for patent ductus arteriosus including closure in adults. Echocardiography. 2015;**32**(Suppl 2):S125-S139

[31] Baumgartner H, Bonhoeffer P, De Groot NM, de Haan F, Deanfield JE, Galie N, et al. ESC Guidelines for the management of grown-up congenital heart disease (new 2010). European Heart Journal. 2010;**31**(23):2915-2957

[32] Wilson W, Taubert KA, Gewitz M, Lockhart PB, Baddour LM, Levison M, et al. Prevention of infective endocarditis: Guidelines from the American Heart Association: A guideline from the American Heart Association Rheumatic Fever, Endocarditis, and Kawasaki Disease Committee, Council on Cardiovascular Disease in the Young, and the Council on Clinical Cardiology, Council on Cardiovascular Surgery and Anesthesia, and the Quality of Care and Outcomes Research Interdisciplinary Working Group. Circulation. 2007;**116**(15):1736-1754

[33] Backer CL, Eltayeb O, Mongé MC, Mazwi ML, Costello JM. Shunt lesions part I: Patent ductus arteriosus, atrial septal defect, ventricular septal defect, and atrioventricular septal defect. Pediatric Critical Care Medicine. 2016;**17**(8 Suppl 1):S302-S309

[34] Prescott S, Keim-Malpass J. Patent ductus arteriosus in the preterm infant. Advances in Neonatal Care. 2017;**17**(1):10-18

[35] Stankowski T, Aboul-Hassan SS, Marczak J, Szymanska A, Augustyn C, Cichon R. Minimally invasive thoracoscopic closure versus thoracotomy in children with patent ductus arteriosus. The Journal of Surgical Research. 2017;**208**(2):1-9

[36] Ozkokeli M, Ates M, Uslu N, Akcar M. Pulmonary and aortic valve endocarditis in an adult patient with silent patent ductus arteriosus. Japanese Heart Journal. 2004;**45**(6): 1057-1056

[37] Balzer DT, Spray TL, McMullin D, Cottingham W, Canter CE. Endarteritis associated with a clinically silent patent ductus arteriosus. American Heart Journal. 1993;**125**(4):1192-1193

[38] Parthenakis FI, Kanakaraki MK, Vardas PE. Images in cardiology: Silent patent ductus arteriosus endarteritis. Heart. 2000;**84**(6):619

[39] Sakai Bizmark R, Chang RR, Tsugawa Y, Zangwill KM, Kawachi I. Impact of AHA's 2007 guideline change on incidence of infective endocarditis in infants and children. American Heart Journal. 2017;**189**(7):110-119

[40] Naik RJ, Patel NR, Wang M, Shah NC. Infective endocarditis prophylaxis: Current practice trend among paediatric cardiologists: Are we following the 2007 guidelines? Cardiology in the Young. 2016;**26**(6):1176-1182

[41] Elsayed YN, Fraser D. Patent ductus arteriosus in preterm infants, Part 1: Understanding the pathophysiologic link between the patent ductus arteriosus and clinical complications. Neonatal Network. 2017;**36**(5):265-272

[42] Boyalla V, Putzu P, Dierckx R, Clark AL, Pellicori P. Patent ductus arteriosus in older adults: Incidental finding or relevant pathology? Journal of the American Geriatrics Society. 2015;**63**(20):409-411

[43] Jacobs AK, Anderson JL, Halperin JL. The evolution and future of ACC/AHA clinical practice guidelines: A 30-year journey: A report of the American College of Cardiology/American Heart Association Task Force on Practice Guidelines. Circulation. 2014;**130**(14):1208-1217. http://circ.ahajournals.org/content/130/14/1208/tab-article-info

Chapter 3

Cardiac Catheterization in Congenital Heart Disease

Neil Tailor, Ranjit Philip and Shyam Sathanandam

Additional information is available at the end of the chapter

http://dx.doi.org/10.5772/intechopen.79981

Abstract

Interventional pediatric cardiology is a specialty of pediatric cardiology that deals specifically with the catheter-based treatment of congenital heart diseases. Cardiac catheterization involves the evaluation and manipulation of the heart and surrounding vessels through catheters place in peripheral vessels. In this chapter we begin by discussing the significant difference between adult and pediatric interventional cardiology. We will discuss basic hemodynamic measurements performed in cardiac catheterization and its application to congenital heart disease. Stent and balloon catheters are briefly discussed. Finally, specific catheter based interventional techniques, indications, and complications for various pediatric congenital heart disease is described.

Keywords: pediatric interventional cardiology, valvuloplasty, angioplasty, balloon catheter, stent

1. Introduction to cardiac catheterization in congenital heart disease

Cardiac catheterization in the pediatric population has similarities with catheterization in adults but very distinct differences. In adults, the primary pathology is isolated coronary atherosclerotic disease, which is exceedingly rare in pediatrics, and valvular disease. The indications, techniques, and interventions performed in pediatrics are different. There are a wide range of therapeutic procedures performed in the pediatric cardiac catheterization lab including device closure of septal defects, balloon angioplasty of stenotic lesions and valvuloplasty of stenotic valves, stenting for vascular stenosis, embolization and device closure of vessels, and even percutaneous pulmonary valve implantation. A complete assessment of the patient is important as well as evaluating and determining the best sedation, vascular access, and potential interventions.

At its most basic, cardiac catheterization is the evaluation and manipulation of the heart and related vessels by catheters placed through peripheral vessels. Most commonly, access is now obtained by the femoral artery and vein using a modified Seldinger technique, which involves placing a sheath and catheter over a wire. Alternative sites include the carotid and jugular, axillary, radial, subclavian, transhepatic, and even umbilical vessels in neonates. Anytime a catheter, wire, or sheath sits in a blood vessel, primarily an artery, there is a risk of occlusion, thromboembolism, and stroke. To prevent this, heparin is routinely administered throughout a catheterization case. Knowledge of basic technique and case-specific complications will help the practitioner in the management of these patients.

2. Basic hemodynamics

Traditionally, cardiac catheterization was the primary tool in the diagnosis and evaluation of congenital heart disease. Before the emergence of echocardiograms, clinical suspicion of congenital heart disease required a cardiac catheterization for definitive diagnosis, possible intervention, and pre-surgical planning. Cardiac catheterization can provide information such as angiographic images by fluoroscopic imaging during contrast injection, pressure measurements, oxygen blood saturations, and estimations of cardiac output and pulmonary vascular resistance. Pressure measurements are taken by way of a fluid-filled pressure transducer attached to a catheter with end-holes that are passed through various vessels and structures in the heart (**Figure 1**). The transducer produces cardiac pressure waveforms that are interpreted by the interventionalist (**Figure 2**). This is especially important in the evaluation of stenosis, diastolic dysfunction, and pulmonary vascular resistance.

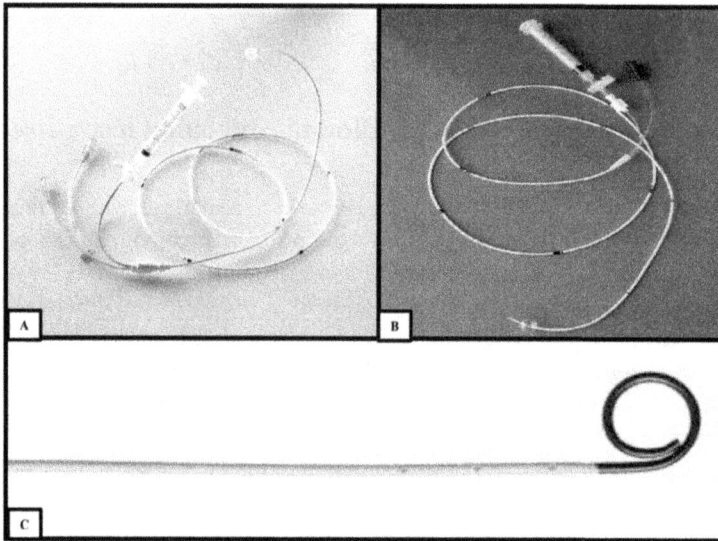

Figure 1. Various cardiac catheters. (A) A thermodilution catheter used to calculate cardiac output. (B) A Berman catheter with an inflatable balloon and side holes is a multiuse catheter. (C) A pigtail multiuse catheter. The multiple side holes allow for angiography of arterial vessels.

In each chamber of the heart, blood can be aspirated through a catheter and a blood oxygen saturation measured. These data can then be used to estimate a patient's cardiac output and ratio of pulmonary blood flow to systemic blood flow (Qp:Qs). In 1870, Adolph Fick described a method for calculating blood flow which was refined and is now known as the Fick Method [1]. Basically, he explained that the release of a substance (in this case, oxygen consumption) in an organ is the product of blood flow across that organ and the concentration difference of a substance (oxygen content difference) proximal and distal to the organ. In other words:

$$\text{Cardiac output} = \frac{\text{Oxygen consumption}}{\text{Oxygen content difference}} \qquad (1)$$

Oxygen consumption is often estimated based on normal values in older children and adults. Oxygen content difference is primarily the product of the change in hemoglobin saturation and the oxygen carrying capacity of hemoglobin (1.36).

$$\text{Oxygen content difference} = 1.36 \times \text{hemoglobin} \times \text{difference in oxygen saturations} \qquad (2)$$

Using this principle, one can estimate the blood flow through any organ by knowing the oxygen blood saturations proximal and distal to the organ and the hemoglobin concentration of blood. In this way, sampling blood in the systemic veins proximal to the heart and blood in the aorta, distal to the heart, can estimate cardiac output. Similarly, sampling blood in the pulmonary arteries and pulmonary veins can estimate pulmonary blood flow.

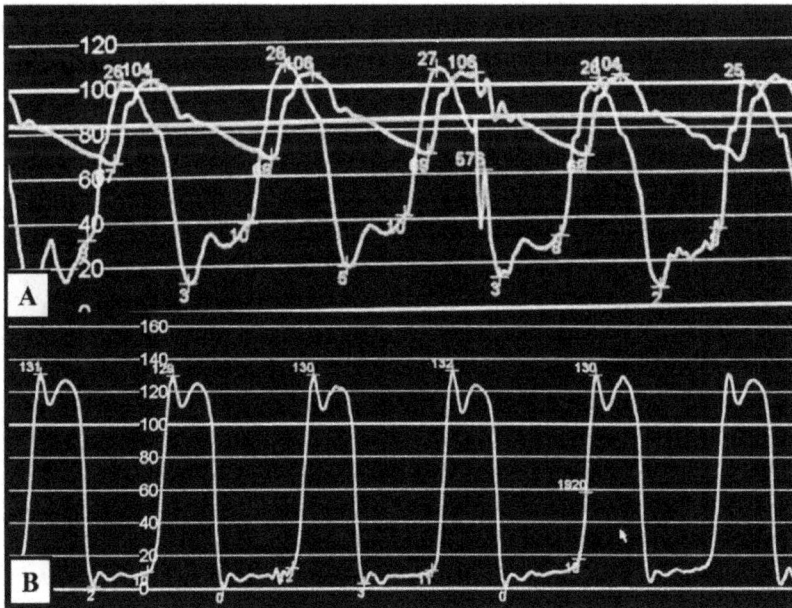

Figure 2. Normal intracardiac pressure tracings in a 10 year old patient. (A) A simultaneous pressure tracing of the right ventricle (red) and the femoral artery (green). (B) Pressure tracing of the left ventricle.

Resistance calculations are then based on Ohm's law of electromagnetism. Georg Ohm was a German born scientist who in 1827 described that the electric current through a conductor is directly proportional to the potential voltage difference divided by the resistance. Modified for body fluid dynamics and a quick variation, it simply states that:

$$\text{Resistance} = \frac{\Delta \text{ Pressure}}{\text{Flow}} \qquad (3)$$

Ohm's law is used to calculate the pulmonary vascular resistance (PVR). The change in pressure across the lungs is estimated by the difference between the left atrial pressure and pulmonary artery pressure in a normal heart. The pulmonary blood flow is estimated by the Fick principle. PVR is an important measure in the diagnosis and management of pulmonary hypertension and pre-surgical planning.

3. Basic interventions

The majority of pediatric cardiac catheterization interventions include balloons, stents, and various devices. The equipment and tools of an interventional cardiologist varies based on experience level and new technological innovations. Attached to a specialized balloon catheter, an inflatable and deflectable balloon is essential in the treatment of stenosis and the deployment of stents. There are a variety of different types of balloons that range in size, shape, and compliance. These specialized balloon catheters have end holes to inflate balloons with contrast solution so they are easily visible on fluoroscopy. Using a specialized device known as a gauge, the balloons are inflated, deflated, and removed from the patient. This is useful in the treatment of vessel stenosis and valve dilation. Balloon interventions carry lesion specific risks described in the subsequent sections of this chapter.

The first intravascular stent use in children was first described in the late 1980s. Indications include those stenotic lesions that are unresponsive to balloon dilation or recur frequently. Additionally, covered stents are using in treating significant tears or aneurysms. Each stent has its own set of characteristics including their size, strength, and "shortening" ability (**Figure 3**). Stents are metal or plastic mesh tubes that are loaded over balloon catheters and expandable

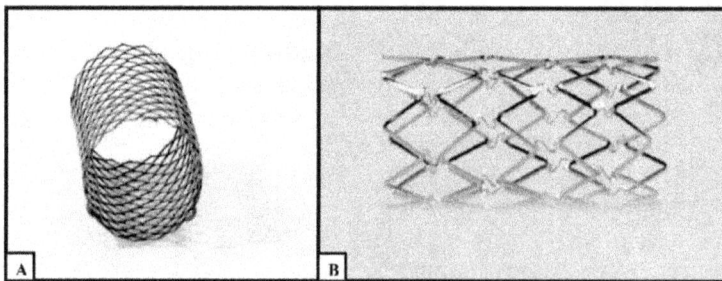

Figure 3. A and B are two different kinds of bare metal stents used in pediatrics. Notice the interconnected mesh wiring and "tube" like shape.

inside a vessel. Covered stents have a surgical fabric-coating that creates a contained tube that is expandable similar to bare stents. Finally, there are a number of devices used to embolize or close vessels and treat septal defects that are described in the following respective sections.

4. Patent ductus arteriosus

4.1. Introduction

The ductus arteriosus is an embryological vessel that connects the systemic and pulmonary circulation and serves to bypass the neonatal lungs. The vessel connects the pulmonary artery to the aortic arch. The patent ductus arteriosus (PDA) is a persistence of the ductus arteriosus after birth. The PDA is useful in cyanotic congenital heart diseases and is kept open until surgical palliation in many cases. This is described further in the chapter on cyanotic congenital heart disease. In the absence of a cyanotic heart lesion, the isolated PDA allows for a portion of oxygenated blood from the left side of the heart to flow back towards the lungs. Isolated PDA accounts for 10% of all congenital heart disease and is unlikely to close naturally in term infants [2]. Long term complications can include congestive heart failure, infective endocarditis, and pulmonary hypertension.

The first closure of the PDA was done by Gross and Hubbard in 1939. The first transcatheter closure of the PDA was performed by Portsmann et al. in 1967 and since then, there have been many developments in the closure of the PDA. Until recently, transcatheter closure of the PDA was not performed in infants less than 5–10 kg, but is now performed in infants as small as 600 g in some centers. Further innovation and experience in this procedure will result in a non-invasive, effective alternative to surgical PDA ligation in nearly all patients.

4.2. Indications

In older patients, the indications for closure of the PDA are well defined. Patients who have signs of left ventricular overload due to the left to right shunting of the PDA should be evaluated for cardiac catheterization closure. A long-standing PDA can lead to congestive left sided heart failure and Eisenmenger's syndrome similar to a ventricular septal defect. The indications for closure in neonates is more controversial. There is currently inadequate data for or against the closure of the PDA in young infants [3], but a general consensus is that transcatheter closure of the PDA in symptomatic infants at 2–3 weeks of age is both safe and effective. Alternatives include surgical ligation and medical closure with a non-steroidal anti-inflammatory drug such as indomethacin or acetaminophen. However, pharmacological treatment of the PDA is effective primarily in premature infants, and has an effective closure rate of around 68% [4].

4.3. Catheterization

Although the procedure is sometimes performed under only echocardiographic guidance and occasionally in the neonatal intensive care unit, we recommend fluoroscopy guidance in the cardiac catheterization lab. Traditionally, both femoral venous and arterial access is

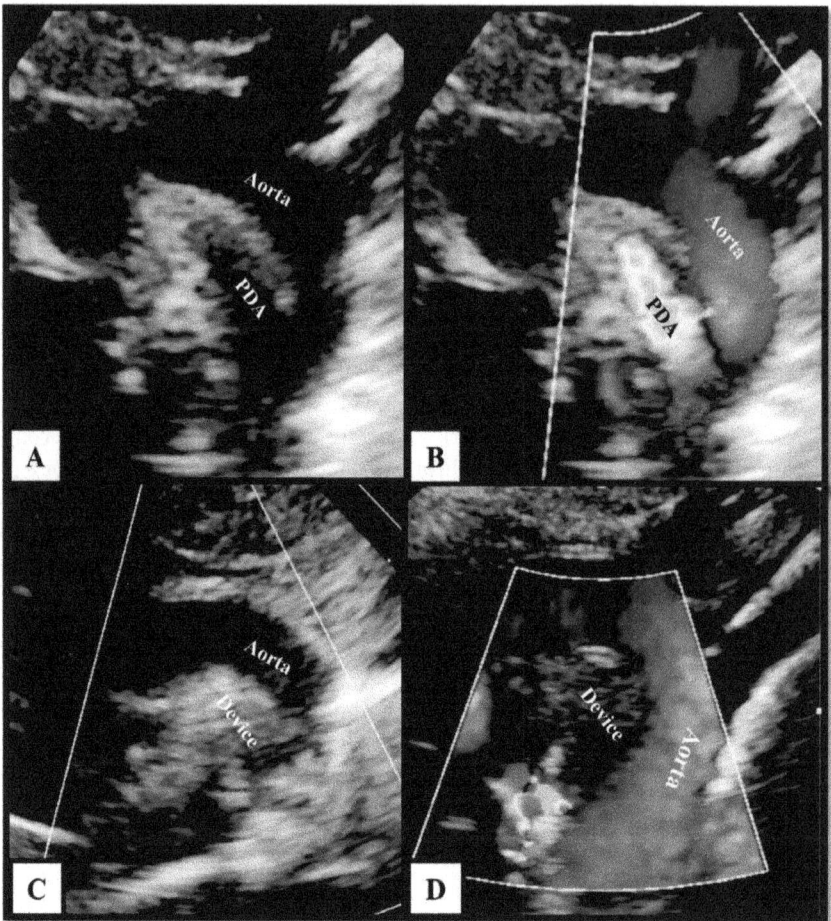

Figure 4. Echocardiographic images of a PDA closure in a 4 week old premature infant who could not be extubated due to pulmonary edema. (A) Two-dimensional (2D) image of the aorta and the PDA as marked. (B) Color Doppler of the aorta and PDA showing opposite flow in each vessel. There is left to right shunting in the PDA. (C and D) After closure with a device, the PDA is no longer visualized by 2D or color Doppler.

obtained. Arterial access is used as a guide for the distal end of the ductus. Recent technique innovation requires only femoral venous access and placement of an esophageal temperature probe. The probe acts as a landmark for the distal end of the ductus. The ductus is engaged by traversing a catheter through the pulmonary artery, ductus, and into the descending aorta.

First, an angiogram is performed to obtain measurements and describe the morphology of the PDA. A PDA with a pulmonary end diameter of less than 2.5 mm can occasionally be closed by coil embolization. These are spring wire coils enmeshed with polyester fibers and delivered through a catheter. The coil occludes the vessel by creating a wire and fabric framework that clots. In most PDAs, an occlusion device is used. A guidewire is used as an anchor and an occlusion device is loaded through a catheter into the PDA. There are various devices used for PDA closure including vascular plugs and two-disk duct occluders similar to atrial septal device occluders. The diameter of the device should be at least the measured diameter of the ductus. Ideally, the device is situated entirely in the ductus arteriosus with no protrusion in either the pulmonary artery or the aorta. Once the device is in position, echocardiography is used to verify no residual shunting, and no obstruction to either the descending aorta or the branch pulmonary arteries. Once this is verified, the device is deployed (**Figures 4–6**).

4.4. Complications

The major complications of the procedure acutely are obstruction of the aorta or branch pulmonary arteries and embolization of the device. The rate of embolization ranges from 1 to 3% and is nearly always retrievable by catheterization without surgical intervention. Loss of distal pulses and vascular injury has been shown to occur in around 20% of premature infants who

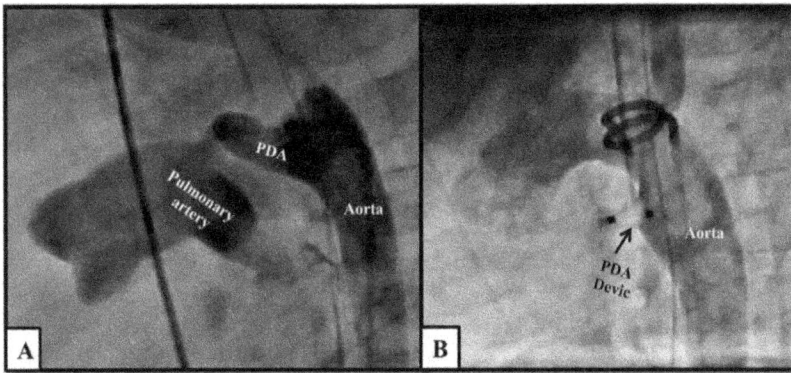

Figure 5. Angiographic images of a PDA closure in a 4 year old patient who presented with left atrial and left ventricular dilation. (A) Contrast injection of the PDA through a pigtail catheter located in the aorta through a retrograde arterial course. (B) Contrast injection angiogram after closure of the duct with visualization of the PDA device. There is no visible stenosis of the aorta.

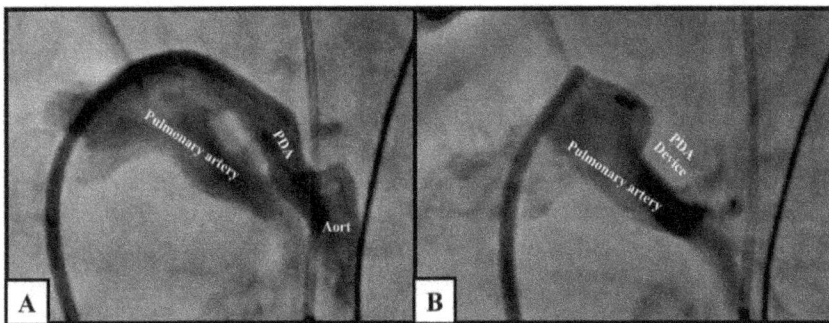

Figure 6. Angiograms of a PDA closure in an 800 g 28 week gestation infant who was unable to wean from ventilatory support. There was no arterial access in this patient. (A) An angiogram performed shows a large PDA similar in morphology to most premature infant ducts. (B) After closure with a microvascular plug device, there is no residual flow through the duct and the left pulmonary artery is unobstructed.

had arterial access [5]. Infants also suffer an entity known as post ligation cardiac syndrome. Six to twelve hours after ligation, these patients suffer a transient low cardiac output state occasionally requiring additional inotropic support. Reported rates are as high as 50% [6].

5. Atrial septal defect

5.1. Introduction

Atrial septal defects (ASD) are holes between the right and left atrium of the heart. Their presence is noted in nearly half of all congenital defects and is important for preserved cardiac output and adequate mixing in a variety of critical congenital heart disease as described in the section on atrial septostomy [7]. Ostium secundum defects are the result of an embryological defect in the septum primum. They are the most common type of ASD with nearly 75% fitting their description. Other types of ASDs include sinus venosus, coronary sinus, or ostium primum defects. Isolated atrial septal defects are typically asymptomatic in infants as the shunting across them is insignificant in early life. Eventually, patients may become symptomatic with frequent respiratory infections, though most are diagnosed due to the presence of a persistent murmur heard by a primary care practitioner and subsequent echocardiogram. Right ventricular and atrial dilation may be present along with a classic fixed split S2 heart sound on auscultation [8].

The first successful surgical closure of an ASD was performed in 1949. It was not until 1972 that the first transcatheter closure of ASDs were performed in animal studies [9]. The first human patient to undergo transcatheter device closure of an ASD was a 17 year old girl in 1975 using a Rashkind foam-covered, six-ribbed device [10]. Since that time, there have been numerous occlusion device revisions and innovations. Since the early 2000s, overall results from transcatheter atrial septal defect device closure have achieved results comparable if not exceeded those of surgical closure [11].

5.2. Indications

As stated before, patients with atrial septal defects rarely have clinically relevant symptoms. Ostium secundum defects are the only type of ASD amenable to device closure. In general, atrial septal defects should be closed in patients with right cardiac chamber enlargement with or without symptoms, a paradoxical embolism, or exercise related cyanosis. Patients who have severe pulmonary arterial hypertension unresponsive to vasodilator therapy, intracardiac thrombus, or a contraindication to antiplatelet agents should not undergo transcatheter closure. Additionally, defects must measure 36 mm or less, have adequate rims, and be located a safe distance from adjacent structures. Those that do not meet these criteria should undergo evaluation for surgical closure.

5.3. Catheterization procedure

All patients should have standard catheterization precautions with general anesthesia, antibiotic prophylaxis, and anti-coagulation with heparin. In particular, patients undergoing this procedure should be started on aspirin before the procedure or be bridged with heparin. A transesophageal echocardiogram (TEE) is typically done simultaneously with the cardiac catheterization to ensure good positioning of the device and no residual defect or obstruction of other valves. Femoral venous percutaneous access is preferred. Arterial access is optional in these cases.

Initially, associated abnormalities including pulmonary venous abnormalities or associated atrial septal defects should be evaluated by TEE. Pressure and flow measurements are first obtained using a Berman or multiuse catheter. The defect is then crossed by a catheter and a wire is positioned in the left upper pulmonary vein through the defect to serve as an anchor. As the septal defects often stretch and are not symmetrical, balloon sizing is regularly performed. A balloon stretched and sized ASD is usually 30% larger than the measured TEE dimension prior to intervention. Balloon sizing also allows for temporary occlusion of the

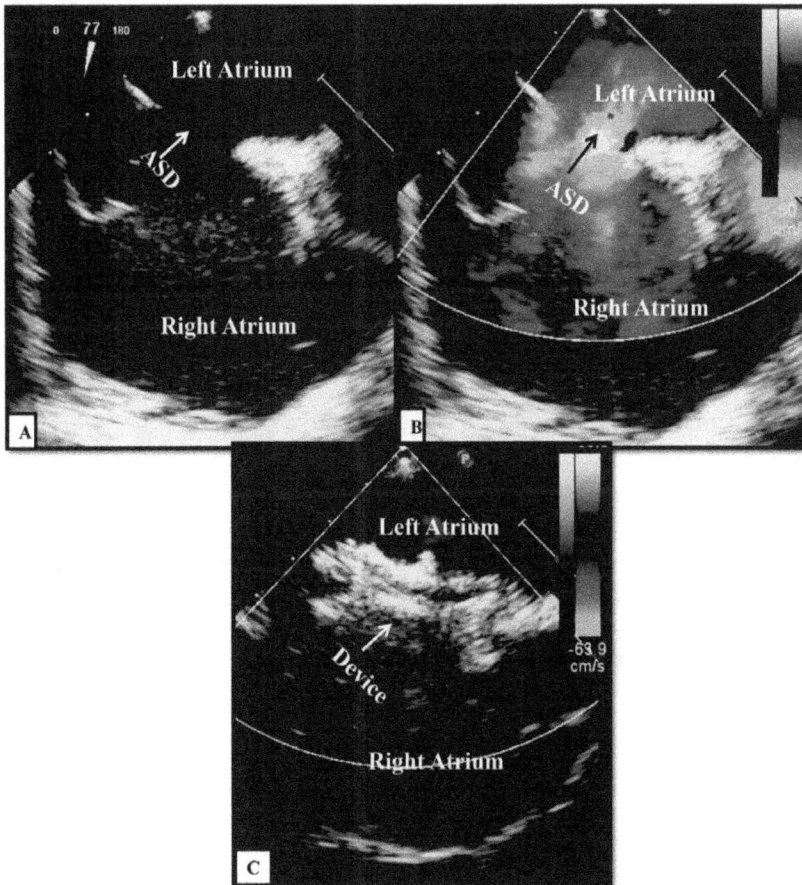

Figure 7. Device closure of an ASD in a 10 y/o asymptomatic patient found to have moderate right atrial and right ventricular dilation. (A) The right atrium is moderately dilated due to a large ostium secundum atrial defect. (B) Color flow demonstrated all left to right shunt (blue color flow in the image). (C) Color Doppler after deployment of a two disk Amplatzer septal occluder shows no residual left to right shunting and complete closure of the ASD.

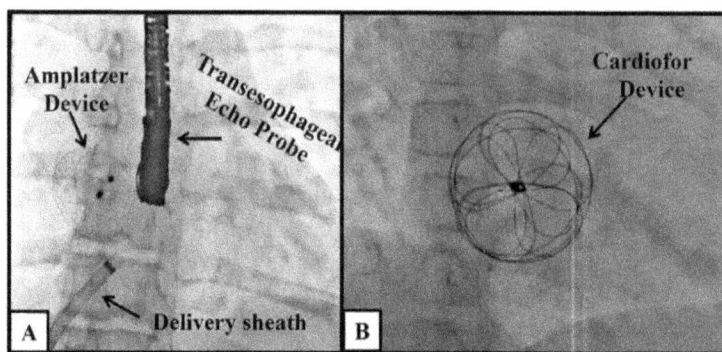

Figure 8. Fluoroscopic images of different deployed ASD closure devices. (A) Amplatzer septal occluder post deployment along with its delivery sheath. ASD closures are typically done under transesophageal echocardiographic guidance. (B) Cardioform septal occluder.

ASD to determine its hemodynamic effects on the heart and whether the patient will tolerate closure. Once this is done, a device is advanced through a sheath to the defect. Most popular devices consist of a two disk system [Gore Helex Septal Occluder (HSO) (W.L. Gore, Flagstaff, AZ) and Amplatzer septal occluder (ASO) (AGA Medical, Golden Valley, MN)]. The distal disk is deployed in the left atrium and pulled back until it is snug against the atrial septum. The proximal disk is then deployed and the device is released (**Figures 7** and **8**). Post procedure repeat chest films and echocardiograms over the next 24 hours are important to verify secure device positioning [12].

5.4. Complications

Reported severe complications in one study was as high as 7%, which is less than that of surgical closure [13]. During deployment of an occlusion device, components rotate and then return to their inherent shape. Device embolization is an unlikely complication but serious complication that occurs in the first 24–48 hours of the procedure. Erosion of a device into the adjacent anterosuperior wall or aorta is 0.1% in the US [14]. Incidence of device-associated thrombus is 1.2% and primarily occurs within the first month of the procedure. For this reason, patients are typically placed on a regimen of aspirin and clopidogrel for 3–6 months. Arrhythmias, primarily atrial fibrillation can occur with any manipulation and scarring of the atrium. The post-procedure incidence of atrial fibrillation is 6% [15]. Additionally, endocarditis prophylaxis is recommended for 6 months after device closure [12].

6. Balloon atrial septostomy

6.1. Introduction and indication

Balloon atrial septostomy, otherwise known as the Rashkind intervention, was described nearly 50 years ago as a life-saving emergent procedure required in particular congenital heart disease. Rashkind first described a transvenous approach for an atrial septostomy in patients with transposition of the great arteries in the early 1960s. The procedure itself involves either widening an existing restrictive atrial level communication (**Figure 9**), or perforating the septum to manufacture a communication. Although the procedure is emergent, it can be planned even before birth based on fetal echocardiography. The primary purpose of an atrial septostomy is to enhance atrial mixing, decompressing the left atrium in a left sided obstructive lesion, or augmenting cardiac output in a right sided obstructed lesion. Primary congenital heart diseases that may require a balloon atrial septostomy include single ventricle physiology such as hypoplastic left heart syndrome and tricuspid atresia, transposition of the great arteries without a ventricular septal defect, and total anomalous pulmonary venous return.

6.2. Catheter procedure

The procedure can be performed in either the intensive care unit or a cardiac catheterization laboratory, the latter being preferred. In some centers, the infants are delivered in the cardiac catheterization lab to avoid any desaturation and cerebral hypoxia from delay. Access may someones be possible through the neonatal umbilical vein. If there are venous duct tortuosities, access through a femoral venous approach is required. Transthoracic echocardiographic guidance is highly recommended. Newborns are too small for a transesophageal echocardiogram. The patient should be anticoagulated with heparin and receive antibiotic prophylaxis at birth.

The procedure begins with advancing a balloon catheter into the right atrium and into the left atrium through the restrictive septum. In some cases, congenital heart disease such as hypoplastic left heart syndrome can have a thick atrial septum without any communication. In this case, a transseptal puncture needle or radiofrequency wire perforation may be required. Once the balloon is in the left atrium, it is inflated and, with a quick short movement, is passed back to the right atrium where it is deflated (**Figure 10**). This procedure is repeated several times and the presence of an atrial shunt is confirmed by echocardiography (**Figure 11**). In rare cases, a stent can be placed in the interatrial communication for a long-lasting result [16].

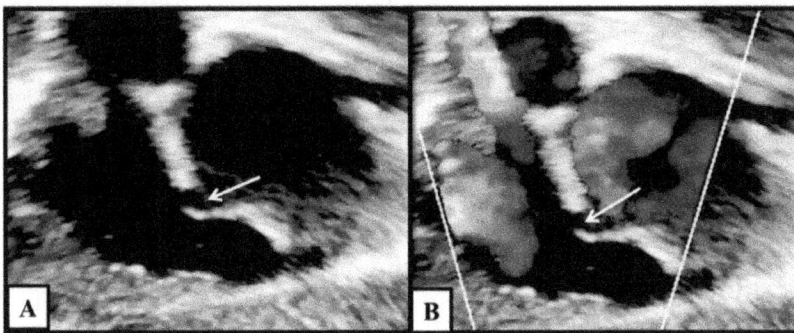

Figure 9. Transthoracic echocardiogram of a term newborn infant with D-transposition of the great vessels and a restrictive atrial septum. (A) 2D image of the restrictive atrial septal defect with bowing of the atrial septum. (B) There is nearly absent color Doppler signal across the defect representing scarce blood flow across the defect.

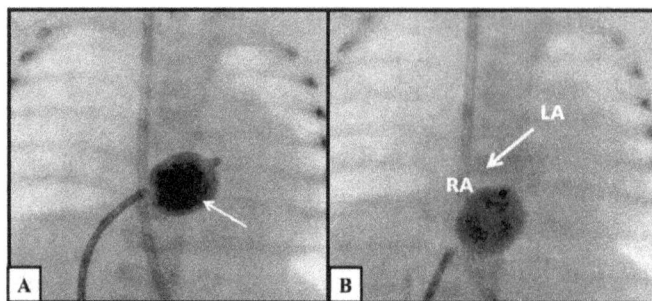

Figure 10. Fluoroscopy of a balloon atrial septostomy in the same patient. (A) The balloon is inflated while positioned in the left atrium with the catheter through the restrictive atrial septal defect. (B) In a swift motion, the inflated balloon is pulled back to the right atrium to dilate the atrial septal defect. This process is repeated a number of times.

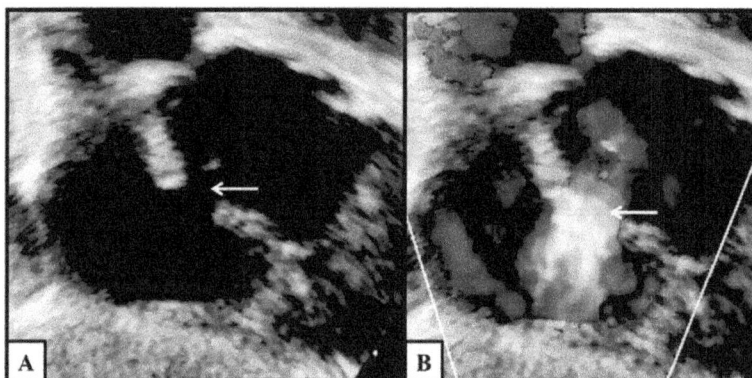

Figure 11. Post atrial septostomy echocardiogram of the same patient. (A) The atrial septal defect has now been dilated. (B) Color Doppler reveals unobstructed left to right shunting across the newly widened defect.

6.3. Complications

Balloon atrial septostomy is a life-saving emergent procedure with rare complications. Rupture of the balloon with embolization of the fragments can occur and require retrieval [17]. Traumatic complications including damage or rupture of the atrial appendage, mitral valve, or pulmonary veins can occur. Stroke has been reported, but recent studies have shown no increase odds of brain injury in patients who undergo a balloon atrial septostomy [18]. The most common complications include transient cardiac arrhythmias that require rapid treatment but generally resolve [16].

7. Coarctation of the aorta

7.1. Introduction

Coarctation of the aorta involves narrowing of various segments of the aorta. This often results in pathologic obstruction of systemic blood flow. Coarctation is the fourth most common congenital heart defect. It comprises of 7% of all congenital heart disease and affects ~0.04% of live births. Males are twice as likely to have coarctation compared to girls [19]. The more severe the narrowing, the more symptomatic a child will be, and the earlier the problem will be noticed. In some cases, coarctation is noted in infancy. In others, however, it may not be noted until school-age or adolescence. Symptoms may include diminished blood pressures in the lower extremities, diminished pulses in the lower extremities, and signs of left sided heart failure including poor feeding, poor weight gain, and cool extremities. In severe cases of coarctation of the aorta, babies may present with hypoxia [20].

Initially, transcatheter balloon angioplasty was introduced in the 1980s as an adjunctive treatment to recurrent coarctation of the aorta following surgical therapy. Both treatments had flaws including re-coarctation of the aorta, residual hypertension, dissection of the aorta, and other aortic wall damage including aneurysm formation [21, 22]. To reduce complications and limitations, balloon-expandable stent therapy was introduced as a novel treatment for congenital heart diseases including coarctation of the aorta in the early 1990s [23]. Since that time, stent therapy has become widely accepted in children and adults for native and re-coarctation of the aorta [24].

7.2. Indications

The primary indication for repair in an older patient is an upper to lower-extremity systolic gradient of greater than 20 mmHg and/or the presence of symptoms including claudication and headaches. Of note, accurate blood pressure measurements are of the utmost importance. Ideally, three consecutive measurements in each extremity is required. Additional criteria include a diameter to diameter ratio of less than 0.6 between the narrowest portion of the coarctation of the abdominal aorta [25]. Cardiac balloon angioplasty and stent placement is rarely performed in small infants presenting with coarctation as rapid growth of the infant results in function coarctation from small stents.

7.3. Catheterization procedure

All patients should have standard catheterization precautions with general anesthesia, antibiotic prophylaxis, and anti-coagulation with heparin. The procedure occurs with a retrograde transfemoral approach by accessing both the femoral artery and vein. Care is taken to access the artery as proximal as possible and to avoid access past the bifurcation of the femoral artery. This ensures access to a large diameter vessel as larger stents require larger sheaths that can increase the risk of vascular compromise of the respective limb.

All patients undergo a complete right and left-heart catheterization as well as a detailed angiogram of the aorta using one of many various angiographic catheters such as a pigtail or multitrack catheter. Rotational angiography can provide additional imaging details of the aorta. Evaluating each branching vessel and its relationship to the coarctation segment is essential. Typically, a stiffer guidewire is positioned across the area of stenosis in preparation for stent placement.

Experience of the interventional cardiologist is of the utmost importance when choosing a stent. Typically, the diameter of the stent should not exceed the abdominal aorta diameter. Additionally, the ratio of the stent diameter to the narrowest coarctation segment should be less than 3.5 [26]. Once the stent is chosen, it is loaded over a balloon-in-balloon catheter. The inner balloon allows repositioning after partial deployment of the stent. Successful treatment is defined as a residual gradient less than 10 mmHg and post intervention vessel caliber of greater than 80% of the normal adjacent aortic segment (**Figure 12**). Per the revised 2015 Bethesda guidelines, patients who have intravascular stent placement should avoid contact sports for 3–6 months post procedure. Patients often require continued antihypertensive medications. They require antiplatelet therapy and endocarditis prophylaxis for up to 6 months post procedure [26].

7.4. Complications and stent/balloon angioplasty versus surgery

Outcomes are generally excellent in the acute and long-term setting. Persistent hypertension is noted in up to 23% of patients requiring continued anti-hypertensive medication. Aortic wall complications are rare but can be severe and lead to cardiovascular compromise. These include dissection and rupture. In a cohort of 565 procedures, there was a 1.6% rate of aortic wall pathology especially in patients who underwent pre-stent angioplasty, balloon angioplasty ratio > 3.5, and age greater than 40 years [27].

Aortic aneurysm is a complication in 5–9%. Most are small and do not require procedural re-intervention, but those that are progressive or large can be treated with placement of a covered stent [27, 28]. Cerebrovascular accidents are exceedingly rare with a rate of less than 1% [29].

Various studies have compared outcomes between surgical repair, balloon angioplasty, and stent placement as treatments for coarctation of the aorta. A study by Forbes et al. compared

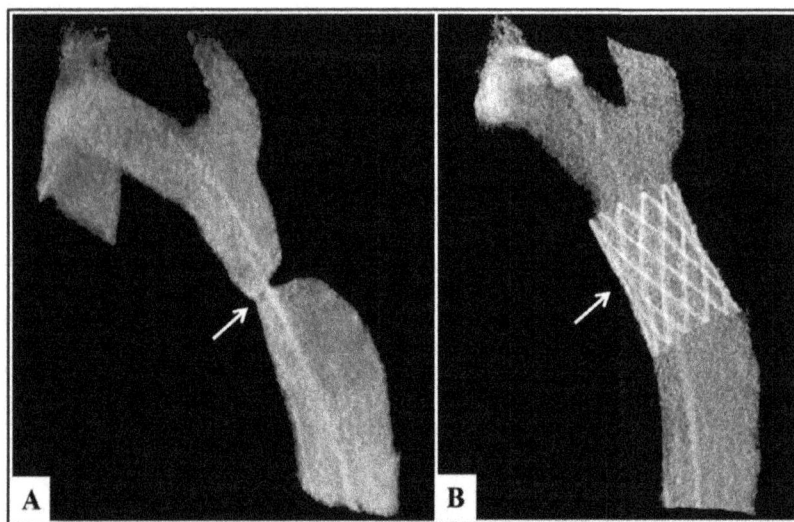

Figure 12. Three-dimensional reconstruction of a rotational angiogram in an 8-year-old boy with severe coarctation of the aorta who underwent stent placement. (A) There is discrete stenosis at the aortic isthmus. A stent loaded balloon catheter can be seen across the narrow portion and into the ascending aorta. (B) Resolution of the angiographic coarctation with placement of a bare metal stent.

intravascular stent placement, balloon angioplasty, and surgical repair in a cohort of 350 patients and found that stent patients had fewer acute complications though at intermediation follow up there was no significant difference in persistent hypertension. There was a significantly higher ratio of the post intervention coarctation are to the adjacent descending aorta and a lower rate of aortic wall injury in the patients with intravascular stents compared to those with balloon angioplasty and surgical repair [25].

8. Aortic stenosis

8.1. Introduction

The aortic valve is a semilunar valve that connects the left ventricle to the aorta in the normal heart. The major difference between the aortic valve and pulmonary valve is the typical absence of an infundibular septum. Aortic stenosis occurs with obstruction below the valve (subvalvar), at the valve (valvar), and above the valve into the left ventricular outflow tract (supravalvar). Aortic stenosis accounts for 3–8% of all congenital heart disease. Valvar stenosis is the most common comprising of 75% of aortic stenosis. Of note, this is typically associated with either a bicuspid valve where two of the 3 cusps are fused, or a unicuspid valve where all three cusps are fused. Aortic stenosis is also associated with various other congenital heart defects as well as genetic syndrome such as Williams syndrome. Symptoms of aortic stenosis are similar to those of any left ventricular outflow tract obstruction including chest pain or syncope with exercise and dyspnea on exertion. There may also be respiratory distress in infants caused by pulmonary edema, though this is typically absent in children and adults [30].

As with most other valvular disease, diagnosis is primarily made by an echocardiogram which is ordered based on clinical suspicion. Echocardiogram can demonstrate the morphology of the valve and characterize the location and degree of obstruction using both continuous wave and pulse wave Doppler, and color Doppler. Untreated aortic stenosis carries with it a 4% risk of endocarditis and a 5% risk of sudden death.

8.2. Indications

Aortic stenosis with less than a transvalvar gradient of 50 mmHg is typically well tolerated. Aortic stenosis is a progressive disease with between 21 and 41% of these patients progressing to severe aortic stenosis defined as a gradient of greater than 50 mmHg. There is an associated 1% per patient-year risk of sudden death in these patients. Balloon aortic valvuloplasty is typically the first line treatment for patients with valvar aortic stenosis with a pressure gradient of greater than 50 mmHg and minimal aortic regurgitation. In patients with subvalvar and supravalvar stenosis, balloon angioplasty is typically not effective. Surgical repair by resection of the areas of stenosis is primarily the treatment for subvalvar and supravalvar stenosis.

8.3. Catheterization procedure

Most patients should have standard catheterization precautions with general anesthesia, antibiotic prophylaxis, and anti-coagulation with heparin. In some cases outside of the neonatal period, the procedure can be performed under conscious sedation. The procedure occurs with a retrograde transfemoral approach by accessing both the femoral artery and vein. Care is taken to access the artery as proximal as possible and to avoid access past the bifurcation of the femoral artery.

This ensures access to a large diameter vessel as larger sheaths that can increase the risk of vascular compromise of the respective limb.

All patients undergo a complete right and left-heart catheterization as well as a detailed angiogram of the aorta and aortic valve. The most important measurement in a transvalvar gradient that can be obtained by a pullback measurement with a catheter, or simultaneous measurements in the aorta and left ventricle using either a trans-atrial-septal approach (in the presence of an ASD or PFO) or an additional arterial access point. The balloon size chosen should be 80–90% of the annulus size to reduce the risk of significant aortic regurgitation.

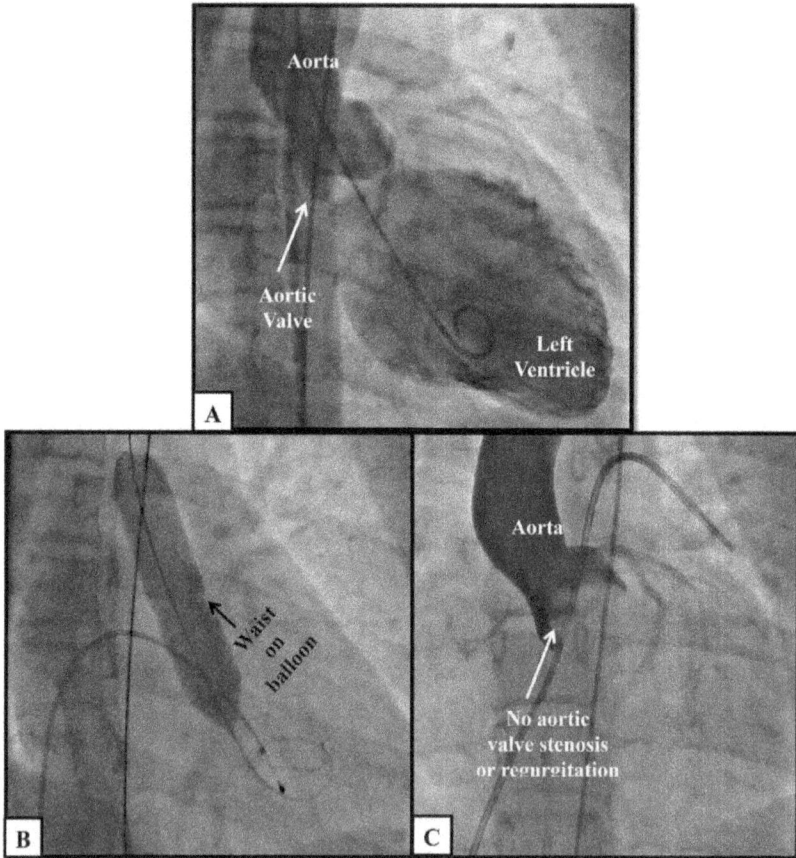

Figure 13. Aortic balloon valvuloplasty in a 14 year old patient with moderate aortic valve stenosis and dizziness. (A) There is moderate stenosis at the level of the aortic valve. A pigtail catheter rests in the left ventricle retrograde from the aorta. (B) During balloon angioplasty of the valve, a "waist" is seen at the area of stenosis. (C) Post valvuloplasty there is no evidence of residual stenosis or aortic regurgitation.

Once the procedure is complete, the gradient is remeasured. Typically, a successful angioplasty results in reducing the gradient by half without a significant increase in aortic regurgitation (**Figure 13**).

8.4. Complications

The most common complications with balloon aortic valvuloplasty are aortic regurgitation and injury to the peripherally accessed vessel. Significant aortic regurgitation occurs in approximately 10% of all aortic valve balloon dilations which is comparable to rates in surgical valvotomy. Oversizing of the aortic balloon to be greater than the size of the aortic valve annulus is a primary risk factor. In patients with balloon ratios greater than 1.0 (I.E. a balloon larger than the diameter of the aortic valve annulus), at least moderate aortic regurgitation is seen in 25% of patients. Vascular injury is less common with improvement in techniques and availability of monitoring equipment [31]. Re-intervention is common and is reportedly required in up to 50% of patients. Typically, each subsequent intervention carries a higher risk of complications. The incidence of moderate aortic regurgitation in repeat dilations is at least 25% [32].

9. Pulmonary stenosis

9.1. Introduction

The pulmonary valve is a semilunar valve that connects the right ventricle to the pulmonary artery in a normal heart. Pulmonary stenosis is primarily a sequelae of congenital heart disease but can be acquired due to surgical or transcatheter interventions. Stenosis can occur at the level of pulmonary valve, above the pulmonary valve, or below the pulmonary valve. Valvular stenosis is the most common, accounting for up to 90% of cases [33]. It is often an isolated finding, but can be associated with congenital heart lesions, most notably tetralogy of Fallot. It is also associated with genetic conditions such as DiGeorge syndrome and 22q11 deletion, Williams syndrome, Alagille syndrome, congenital rubella, and Noonan's syndrome. Noonan syndrome is particularly important as it results in dysplastic, thickened pulmonary valve leaflets that typically do not respond well to catheter-based balloon valvuloplasty. Patients with tetralogy of Fallot are more likely to have a component of sub-valvar and infundibular stenosis [34].

Patients with mild isolated pulmonary stenosis are typically asymptomatic and the stenosis rarely progresses rapidly. Symptoms are associated with the resulting decrease in cardiac output from stenosis. These include dyspnea on exertion, fatigue, and right ventricular hypertrophy, right ventricular diastolic and systolic dysfunction. Patients with severe pulmonary stenosis in the neonatal or early childhood can present with cyanosis in the setting of a intracardiac shunt such as an atrial septal defect.

Diagnoses by echocardiogram is the gold standard. Two-dimensional and three-dimensional echocardiography can evaluate the morphology of the stenosis and pulmonary valve, and evaluate the function and size of the right ventricle. Continuous and pulse wave Doppler can help determine pressure gradients and color Doppler can help quantify and resultant pulmonary regurgitation. In some cases, MRI can accurately assess the degree of regurgitation, flow across the valve, and measure right ventricular size [35].

The three main treatment modalities for pulmonary valve stenosis are balloon pulmonary valvuloplasty, surgical valvotomy, and pulmonary valve replacement, either by surgery or cardiac catheterization. The first balloon valvuloplasty of the pulmonary valve was done in 1979 and is by far the procedure of choice. Valvuloplasty is generally safe and effective in greater than 90% of patients [36].

9.2. Indications

Balloon pulmonary valvuloplasty is indicated for asymptomatic patients with a domed valve morphology, a peak gradient by echocardiography of greater than 60 mmHg, and up to moderate pulmonary regurgitation. Symptomatic patients are treated with an echocardiographic gradient of greater than 50 mmHg and less than moderate pulmonary regurgitation. Immediate effects of balloon valvuloplasty include improved longitudinal right ventricular motion, reduced dyssynchrony in pediatric patients, reduction of tricuspid regurgitation, and improvement in the pulmonary valve gradient. Patients with supravalvar and subvalvar pulmonary stenosis may undergo balloon valvuloplasty but is often less effective, primarily in patients with Noonan syndrome.

9.3. Catheterization procedure

All patients should have standard catheterization precautions with general anesthesia, antibiotic prophylaxis, and anti-coagulation with heparin. Percutaneous femoral venous access is the preferred entry site for balloon pulmonary valvuloplasty. The procedure begins with pressure measurements of the right ventricular and pulmonary artery using a Berman or other multipurpose catheter. Pulmonary valve are can be calculated using the Gorlin formula. Simultaneous recording of the right ventricle and femoral artery pressure is done to assess severity of the obstruction. If the right ventricular systolic pressure is greater than 75% of the systemic systolic pressure, there is significant pulmonary valve obstruction. Angiography is an important tool in confirming the site of stenosis in addition to obtaining accurate measurements of the pulmonary valve annulus [37].

A guidewire is positioned in the distal left pulmonary or right pulmonary artery. In infants, the wire may be positioned in the descending aorta through the patent ductus arteriosus. The purpose of the wire is to guide the balloon catheter and increase its stability. A number of different balloon catheters are available and are often chosen based on availability and experience of the interventional cardiologist. The diameter of the balloon should be 1.2–1.4 times the size of the pulmonary valve annulus with a recommended ratio of 1.2–1.25 [38]. In cases of a dysplastic pulmonary valve, as is typically found in Noonan's syndrome, a ratio of 1.4–1.5 may be used [39]. Successful balloon valvuloplasty is defined as a residual gradient of less than 30 mmHg. Patients with successful valvuloplasty may return to competitive sports 3–6 months post procedure (**Figures 14 and 15**).

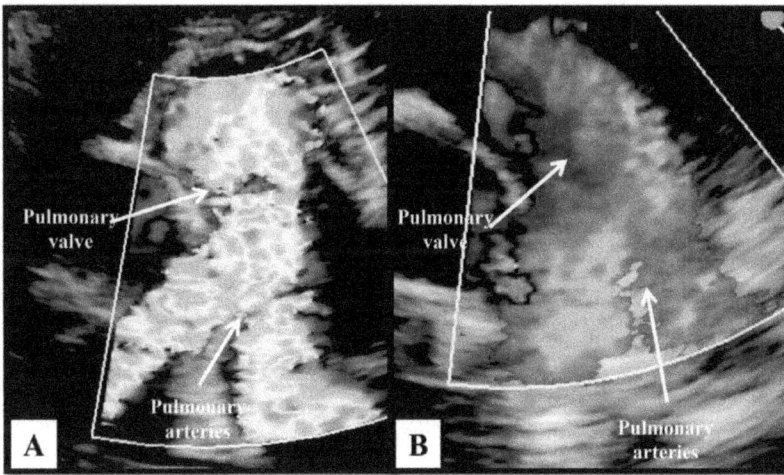

Figure 14. Color Doppler transthoracic echocardiogram of a 2 year old patient with trisomy 21 and pulmonary stenosis who underwent balloon pulmonic valvuloplasty. (A) There is flow acceleration (blue and red color speckling) across the pulmonary valve indicating valvar stenosis. (B) Post balloon pulmonic valvuloplasty there is no flow acceleration or signs of obstruction.

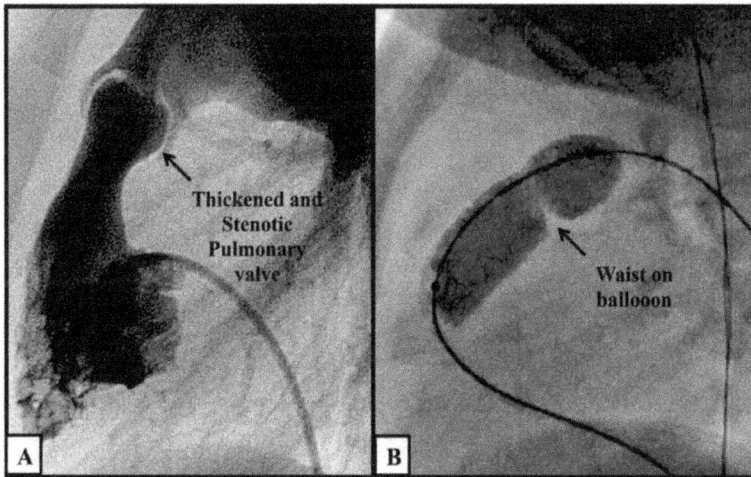

Figure 15. Fluoroscopic images of the above patient during a balloon pulmonic valvuloplasty. (A) There is a thickened and stenotic pulmonary valve typical of patients with Noonan syndrome. (B) During balloon valvuloplasty a "waist" at the area of stenosis is seen.

9.4. Complications

Severe complications are rare occurring in 0.6% of cases and mortality in 0.2% [40]. A major complication is transient but severe right ventricular outflow tract obstruction (sometimes known as a "suicide right ventricle") that can occur immediately after valvuloplasty. Long standing or severe pulmonary stenosis results in right ventricular hypertrophy. When the stenosis is resolved and the systolic right ventricular pressure drops, the hypertrophy results in acute narrowing of the outflow chamber and must be treated with fluid resuscitation and beta blockade [41].

The most common long term side effect is pulmonary regurgitation and recurrent pulmonary stenosis [42]. One study found that 60% of patients followed for 10 years after pulmonary valvuloplasty had at least moderate pulmonary regurgitation. However, pulmonary regurgitation was well tolerated in the majority of patients. Only 5% had right ventricular dysfunction and 3% required intervention [43]. The lower the balloon:annulus ratio, the less risk of significant pulmonary regurgitation. The Long term impact of chronic pulmonary regurgitation from pulmonary valvuloplasty is not well studied. Surrogate data from pulmonary regurgitation secondary to surgical valvotomy or valvectomy suggests that right ventricular function begins to deteriorate after the first several decades [44].

Restenosis occurs in up to 25% of patients who undergo valvuloplasty defined as a peak gradient of >36 mmHg in 1–2 years post procedure. Around 15% of patients who have restenosis will require re-intervention with either surgery or repeat balloon pulmonary valvuloplasty. Risk factors for recurrent stenosis include a dysplastic valve, small annulus, high initial gradient, and a small balloon:annulus ratio defined as less than 1.2 [45].

Author details

Neil Tailor, Ranjit Philip and Shyam Sathanandam*

*Address all correspondence to: ssathan2@uthsc.edu

Le Bonheur Children's Hospital, University of Tennessee, Memphis, TN, USA

References

[1] Fick A. Ueber die Messung dea Blutquantums in den Herzventrikela. Seitung der Physikalisches und Medicinisches Gesellschaft zu Würzburg. 1970;2:290-291

[2] Donti A, Formigari R, Bonvicini M, Prandstraller D, Bronzetti G, Picchio FM. Transcatheter closure of the patent ductus arteriosus with new-generation devices: Comparative data and follow-up results. Italian Heart Journal: Official Journal of the Italian Federation of Cardiology. 2002;3:122-127

[3] Bose CL, Laughon MM. Patent ductus arteriosus: Lack of evidence for common treatments. Archives of Disease in Childhood Fetal and Neonatal Edition. 2007;92:F498-F502. DOI: 10.1136/adc.2005.092734

[4] Mitra S, Florez ID, Tamayo ME, Mbuagbaw L, Vanniyasingam T, Veroniki AA, et al. Association of placebo, indomethacin, ibuprofen, and acetaminophen with closure of

hemodynamically significant patent ductus arteriosus in preterm infants: A systematic review and meta-analysis. Journal of the American Medical Association. 2018;**319**: 1221-1238. DOI: 10.1001/jama.2018.1896

[5] Backes CH, Cheatham SL, Deyo GM, Leopold S, Ball MK, Smith CV, et al. Percutaneous patent ductus arteriosus (PDA) closure in very preterm infants: Feasibility and complications. Journal of the American Heart Association: Cardiovascular and Cerebrovascular Disease. 2016;**5**:e002923. DOI: 10.1161/JAHA.115.002923

[6] El-Khuffash AF, Jain A, Weisz D, Mertens L, McNamara PJ. Assessment and treatment of post patent ductus arteriosus ligation syndrome. The Journal of Pediatrics. 2014;**165**: 46-52.e1. DOI: 10.1016/j.jpeds.2014.03.048

[7] Rodriguez FH 3rd, Moodie DS, Parekh DR, Franklin WJ, Morales DL, Zafar F, et al. Outcomes of hospitalization in adults in the United States with atrial septal defect, ventricular septal defect, and atrioventricular septal defect. The American Journal of Cardiology. 2011;**108**:290-293. DOI: 10.1016/j.amjcard.2011.03.036

[8] Geva T, Martins JD, Wald RM. Atrial septal defects. Lancet (London, England). 2014;**383**:1921-1932. DOI: 10.1016/s0140-6736(13)62145-5

[9] King T, Mills N, King N. A history of ASD closure. Cardiac Interventions Today. October 2010. ISSN 2572-5955 print and ISSN 2572-5963 online

[10] King TD, Thompson SL, Steiner C, Mills NL. Secundum atrial septal defect. Nonoperative closure during cardiac catheterization. Journal of the American Medical Association. 1976;**235**:2506-2509

[11] Suchon E, Pieculewicz M, Tracz W, Przewlocki T, Sadowski J, Podolec P. Transcatheter closure as an alternative and equivalent method to the surgical treatment of atrial septal defect in adults: Comparison of early and late results. Medical Science Monitor: International Medical Journal of Experimental and Clinical Research. 2009;**15**:Cr612-Cr617

[12] Vasquez AF, Lasala JM. Atrial septal defect closure. Cardiology Clinics. 2013;**31**:385-400. DOI: 10.1016/j.ccl.2013.05.003

[13] Du ZD, Hijazi ZM, Kleinman CS, Silverman NH, Larntz K. Comparison between transcatheter and surgical closure of secundum atrial septal defect in children and adults: Results of a multicenter nonrandomized trial. Journal of the American College of Cardiology. 2002;**39**:1836-1844

[14] Divekar A, Gaamangwe T, Shaikh N, Raabe M, Ducas J. Cardiac perforation after device closure of atrial septal defects with the Amplatzer septal occluder. Journal of the American College of Cardiology. 2005;**45**:1213-1218. DOI: 10.1016/j.jacc.2004.12.072

[15] Giardini A, Donti A, Sciarra F, Bronzetti G, Mariucci E, Picchio FM. Long-term incidence of atrial fibrillation and flutter after transcatheter atrial septal defect closure in adults. International Journal of Cardiology. 2009;**134**:47-51. DOI: 10.1016/j.ijcard.2008.02.003

[16] Cinteza E, Carminati M. Balloon atrial septostomy—Almost half a century after. Maedica. 2013;**8**:280-284

[17] El-Said HG, Ing FF, Grifka RG, Nihill MR, Morris C, Getty-Houswright D, et al. 18-year experience with transseptal procedures through baffles, conduits, and other intra-atrial patches. Catheterization and Cardiovascular Interventions: Official Journal of the Society for Cardiac Angiography & Interventions. 2000;**50**:434-439 discussion 40

[18] Applegate SE, Lim DS. Incidence of stroke in patients with d-transposition of the great arteries that undergo balloon atrial septostomy in the University Healthsystem Consortium Clinical Data Base/Resource Manager. Catheterization and Cardiovascular Interventions: Official Journal of the Society for Cardiac Angiography & Interventions. 2010;**76**:129-131. DOI: 10.1002/ccd.22463

[19] Talner CN. Report of the New England regional infant cardiac program, by Donald C, Fyler MD. Pediatrics, 1980;**65**(suppl):375-461. Pediatrics. 1998;**102**:258-259. http://pediatrics.aappublications.org/content/pediatrics/102/Supplement_1/258.full.pdf

[20] Malcic I, Kniewald H, Jelic A, Saric D, Bartonicek D, Dilber D, et al. Coarctation of the aorta in children in the 10-year epidemiological study: Diagnostic and therapeutic consideration. Lijecnicki Vjesnik. 2015;**137**:9-17

[21] Rao PS, Galal O, Smith PA, Wilson AD. Five-to nine-year follow-up results of balloon angioplasty of native aortic coarctation in infants and children. Journal of the American College of Cardiology. 1996;**27**:462-470

[22] Hager A, Schreiber C, Nutzl S, Hess J. Mortality and restenosis rate of surgical coarctation repair in infancy: A study of 191 patients. Cardiology. 2009;**112**:36-41. DOI: 10.1159/000137697

[23] O'Laughlin MP, Perry SB, Lock JE, Mullins CE. Use of endovascular stents in congenital heart disease. Circulation. 1991;**83**:1923-1939

[24] Weber HS, Cyran SE. Endovascular stenting for native coarctation of the aorta is an effective alternative to surgical intervention in older children. Congenital Heart Disease. 2008;**3**:54-59. DOI: 10.1111/j.1747-0803.2007.00148.x

[25] Forbes TJ, Kim DW, Du W, Turner DR, Holzer R, Amin Z, et al. Comparison of surgical, stent, and balloon angioplasty treatment of native coarctation of the aorta: An observational study by the CCISC (Congenital Cardiovascular Interventional Study Consortium). Journal of the American College of Cardiology. 2011;**58**:2664-2674. DOI: 10.1016/j.jacc.2011.08.053

[26] Forbes TJ, Gowda ST. Intravascular stent therapy for coarctation of the aorta. Methodist DeBakey Cardiovascular Journal. 2014;**10**:82-87 https://www.ncbi.nlm.nih.gov/pmc/articles/PMC4117325/pdf/MDCVJ-10-082.pdf

[27] Forbes TJ, Garekar S, Amin Z, Zahn EM, Nykanen D, Moore P, et al. Procedural results and acute complications in stenting native and recurrent coarctation of the aorta in patients over 4 years of age: A multi-institutional study. Catheterization and Cardiovascular Interventions: Official Journal of the Society for Cardiac Angiography & Interventions. 2007;**70**:276-285. DOI: 10.1002/ccd.21164

[28] Qureshi AM, McElhinney DB, Lock JE, Landzberg MJ, Lang P, Marshall AC. Acute and intermediate outcomes, and evaluation of injury to the aortic wall, as based on 15 years experience of implanting stents to treat aortic coarctation. Cardiology in the Young. 2007;**17**:307-318. DOI: 10.1017/s1047951107000339

[29] Holzer R, Qureshi S, Ghasemi A, Vincent J, Sievert H, Gruenstein D, et al. Stenting of aortic coarctation: Acute, intermediate, and long-term results of a prospective multi-institutional registry—Congenital Cardiovascular Interventional Study Consortium (CCISC). Catheterization and Cardiovascular Interventions: Official Journal of the Society for Cardiac Angiography & Interventions. 2010;**76**:553-563. DOI: 10.1002/ccd.22587

[30] Schneider DJMJ. Aortic stenosis. In: Allen HDDD, Shaddy RE, Feltes TF, editors. Moss and Adams' Heart Disease in Infants, Children, and Adolescents: Including the Fetus and Young Adult. 7th ed. Philadelphia, PA: Lippincott Williams & Wilkins; 2008. pp. 968-987

[31] Pedra CA, Sidhu R, McCrindle BW, Nykanen DG, Justo RN, Freedom RM, et al. Outcomes after balloon dilation of congenital aortic stenosis in children and adolescents. Cardiology in the Young. 2004;**14**:315-321. DOI: 10.1017/s1047951104003105

[32] Satou GM, Perry SB, Lock JE, Piercey GE, Keane JF. Repeat balloon dilation of congenital valvar aortic stenosis: Immediate results and midterm outcome. Catheterization and Cardiovascular Interventions: Official Journal of the Society for Cardiac Angiography & Interventions. 1999;**47**:47-51. DOI: 10.1002/(sici)1522-726x(199905)47:1<47::aid-ccd10>3.0.co;2-o

[33] Driscoll DJ, Michels VV, Gersony WM, Hayes CJ, Keane JF, Kidd L, et al. Occurrence risk for congenital heart defects in relatives of patients with aortic stenosis, pulmonary stenosis, or ventricular septal defect. Circulation. 1993;**87**:I114-I120

[34] Fathallah M, Krasuski RA. Pulmonic valve disease: Review of pathology and current treatment options. Current Cardiology Reports. 2017;**19**:108. DOI: 10.1007/s11886-017-0922-2

[35] Saremi F, Gera A, Ho SY, Hijazi ZM, Sanchez-Quintana D. CT and MR imaging of the pulmonary valve. Radiographics: A Review Publication of the Radiological Society of North America, Inc. 2014;**34**:51-71. DOI: 10.1148/rg.341135026

[36] Kan JS, White RI Jr, Mitchell SE, Gardner TJ. Percutaneous balloon valvuloplasty: A new method for treating congenital pulmonary-valve stenosis. The New England Journal of Medicine. 1982;**307**:540-542. DOI: 10.1056/nejm198208263070907

[37] Rao PS. Percutaneous balloon pulmonary valvuloplasty: State of the art. Catheterization and Cardiovascular Interventions: Official Journal of the Society for Cardiac Angiography & Interventions. 2007;**69**:747-763. DOI: 10.1002/ccd.20982

[38] Garty Y, Veldtman G, Lee K, Benson L. Late outcomes after pulmonary valve balloon dilatation in neonates, infants and children. The Journal of Invasive Cardiology. 2005;**17**:318-322 http://europepmc.org/abstract/MED/16003007

[39] Rao PS. Balloon dilatation in infants and children with dysplastic pulmonary valves: Short-term and intermediate-term results. American Heart Journal. 1988;**116**:1168-1173

[40] Stanger P, Cassidy SC, Girod DA, Kan JS, Lababidi Z, Shapiro SR. Balloon pulmonary valvuloplasty: Results of the valvuloplasty and angioplasty of congenital anomalies registry. The American Journal of Cardiology. 1990;**65**:775-783

[41] Fawzy ME, Galal O, Dunn B, Shaikh A, Sriram R, Duran CM. Regression of infundibular pulmonary stenosis after successful balloon pulmonary valvuloplasty in adults. Catheterization and Cardiovascular Diagnosis. 1990;**21**:77-81

[42] Merino-Ingelmo R, Santos-de Soto J, Coserria-Sánchez F, Descalzo-Señoran A, Valverde-Pérez I. Long-term results of percutaneous balloon valvuloplasty in pulmonary valve stenosis in the pediatric population. Revista Española de Cardiología (English Edition). 2014;**67**:374-379. DOI: 10.1016/j.rec.2013.08.020

[43] Devanagondi R, Peck D, Sagi J, Donohue J, Yu S, Pasquali SK, et al. Long-term outcomes of balloon valvuloplasty for isolated pulmonary valve stenosis. Pediatric Cardiology. 2017;**38**:247-254. DOI: 10.1007/s00246-016-1506-4

[44] Earing MG, Connolly HM, Dearani JA, Ammash NM, Grogan M, Warnes CA. Long-term follow-up of patients after surgical treatment for isolated pulmonary valve stenosis. Mayo Clinic Proceedings. 2005;**80**:871-876. DOI: 10.4065/80.7.871

[45] Rao PS, Galal O, Patnana M, Buck SH, Wilson AD. Results of three to 10 year follow up of balloon dilatation of the pulmonary valve. Heart (British Cardiac Society). 1998;**80**: 591-595

Impact of Modified Ultrafiltration in Congenital Heart Disease Patients Treated with Cardiopulmonary Bypass

Pedro José Curi-Curi, Elizabeth Aguilar Alanis,

Juan Calderón-Colmenero,

Jorge Luis Cervantes-Salazar,

Rodrigo Reyes Pavón and

Samuel Ramírez-Marroquín

Additional information is available at the end of the chapter

http://dx.doi.org/10.5772/intechopen.80599

Abstract

Modified ultrafiltration is used in cardiac surgery with cardiopulmonary bypass in order to diminish systemic inflammatory response syndrome. We aimed to show its utility for removing pro-inflammatory agents in operated pediatric patients with congenital heart disease and its impact at operative care. A clinical case control trial was designed, including patients with simple congenital heart disease operated on with cardiopulmonary bypass in a 1-year period. We randomized them to a problematic group (with modified ultrafiltration, n = 15) and a control group (without it, n = 16), and blood samples to measure interleukins (6 and 10), 3d and 4d complement fraction concentrations were taken at the following times: baseline, before cardiopulmonary bypass, after it, after modified ultrafiltration, and from the ultrafiltration concentrate. Operative clinical end points of success were defined as hemodynamic stability, absence of morbidity, and lack of mortality. We observed a higher significant interleukin six concentration in the problematic group patients at baseline, as well as a higher removal of this pro-inflammatory agent at the ultrafiltration concentrate. Modified ultrafiltration has a positive impact over simple congenital heart disease surgery with cardiopulmonary bypass because of removing interleukin 6. We recommend its routinely use when hemodynamic conditions are favorable.

Keywords: cardiopulmonary bypass, congenital heart disease, interleukin

1. Introduction

Cardiopulmonary bypass (CPB) allowed the correction of several congenital heart diseases such as intracardiac malformations, but it is well known that this is not a harmless procedure because it can lead to a systemic inflammatory response syndrome (SIRS), with activation of complement, cytokines, coagulation, and fibrinolysis pathways. Factors that contribute to the development of SIRS include blood contact with the synthetic surface of cardiopulmonary bypass components, as well as leukocyte and endothelial activation after tissue ischemia and reperfusion [1–5]. If there is a severe inflammatory response, it could also develop a multiorgan dysfunction syndrome that increases morbidity and mortality of the patients at pediatric intensive care units (PICUs). Some of the methods used to quantify the magnitude of SRIS due to the use of CPB include measurement of blood cytokine concentrations (interleukins 1 and 6), complement activation products (C3d and C4d), and also coagulation activated factors (Von Willebrand, fibrinogen, and factor VIII) [6].

There are several operative strategies for diminishing SRIS and its clinical repercussion, such as the use of steroids, modified tubular surfaces for CPB, and ultrafiltration. Despite the single or combined use of these strategies [7–12], ultrafiltration is the one that probably removes a larger amount of pro-inflammatory agents, as well as water (volume) [13]. The two ultrafiltration technique modalities widely accepted for pediatric cardiac surgery are conventional ultrafiltration (CUF) and modified ultrafiltration (MUF). CUF is applied in CPB during the heart re-warming period and MUF right after ending CPB.

Currently, there is no enough evidence that favor routinely use of MUF [14–19], and we can still find some controversies regarding the benefits of this technique [20–22]. Additionally, most reports of the literature are focalized in adult cohorts of patients, and there is few information provided for pediatric population that shows the real impact of MUF in the remotion of pro-inflammatory agents due to CPB use. Therefore, we aimed to study the real utility of MUF for remotion of pro-inflammatory agents induced by CPB in operated pediatric patients with simple congenital heart disease. We made a special emphasis in hemodynamic variables, morbidity and mortality at the operative period.

2. Material and methods

2.1. Study design

A prospective, randomized, analytic, clinical case-control trial was designed at the Department of Pediatric Cardiac and Congenital Heart Surgery of a single center during a 1-year period of time. Inclusion criteria were: age ≤ 18 years and simple congenital heart disease that required elective surgical treatment with CPB use for at least 30 minutes. Exclusion criteria were preoperative renal failure, preoperative cardiogenic shock requiring the use of inotropes, preoperative sepsis, preoperative mechanical ventilatory support ≤48 hours, preoperative lactate concentration ≥ 3 mmol/L, and cardiac reoperation. Patients were randomized in two study groups: problematic group (with MUF) and control group (without MUF). With the use of an electronic URNA software, a statistical person randomized the patients and told the perfusionist who was the only surgical team person informed about the results of randomization. All patients included in this study were operated on with informed consent signed by their parents or tutors. The study was also approved by our institutional research and ethics committee.

2.2. Modified ultrafiltration (MUF) technique

Patients randomized to problematic group (with MUF), when informed to the perfusionist, were prepared for CPB with an additional MUF set. Once CPB was ended and hemodynamic stability of the patient was provided, the surgeon was told not to remove the venous cannula, and the venous line was clamped just before its connection to the reservoir. Arterial and venous line pathways were released in order to begin MUF with a 10–20 ml/kg/min flow. MUF continuous flow was achieved pumping the venous residual reservoir volume by means of the arterial line to the patient. A 150–200 mmHg venous vacuum was applied when needed. MUF lasted 10–20 minutes in order to reach a desired hematocrit level and obtain a suitable volume and electrolyte balance. MUF was stopped in case of hemodynamic instability. Once ended, MUF volume was restored to the patient from the hemofilter and venous cannula, allowing the surgeon for decannulation of the patient.

2.3. Biochemical and clinical operative analysis

Biochemical and clinical results were compared between the two study groups at the operative period. Biochemical results were the concentration of cytokine (interleukin 6 and 10) and complement activated products (C3d and C4d). These concentrations were measured from blood samples at the following times: T0 (baseline, at the beginning of anesthesia induction), T1 (before CPB), T2 (immediately after CPB), and T3 (immediately after MUF, in the problem group). The same agents were measured in the MUF fluid concentrate of the problematic group after the procedure (T4). Clinical operative results were evaluated in terms of hemodynamic instability (>20% post-CPB variation respect to previous CPB values of at least three of the following five hemodynamic variables: heart rate, systolic, diastolic and mean blood pressure, and central venous pressure), operative morbidity, and mortality. Operative clinical end points of success were defined as hemodynamic stability, absence of morbidity, and lack of mortality.

2.4. Laboratory analysis of the fluid samples

All patient samples were obtained from central or peripheral blood and collected in tubes without heparin (vacutainer, Becton Dickinson). A 3-ml blood sample was obtained for each of the study times (T0, T1, T2, and T3). The same volume of T4 samples were obtained from the ultrafiltration fluid concentrate. All of the samples were centrifugated at 3000 rpm during 15 minutes, 4°C, and cryopreserved in aliquots of 1.5 ml at −75°C. Interleukin concentrations (IL-6 and IL-10) were measured by means of an ELISA sandwich technique with the use of monoclonal antibodies (PeproTech, New Jersey, EUA). Complement activation products (C3d and C4d) were measured with the same technique, using commercial kits (Bachem, San

Carlos, CA, EUA). Optical density was determined at 450 nm in the ELISA plate detector. Concentrations of IL-6, IL-10 (pg/ml) as well as C3d and C4d (ng/ml) were calculated by means of a GraphPad Software v. 4.2.

2.5. Statistical analysis

Information was registered in evaluation sheets, stored in an electronic Excel page, and analyzed by means of a Prisma Graphics v 3.1 statistical software. Continuous variables are presented as a mean, standard deviation, and variability ranges (minimum and maximum). Categorical data are presented by means of frequency and percentages in relation to the population at risk. Comparison between the two study groups was made by means of a Student t test for continuous variables. A chi-square (χ^2) test was used for comparing categorical variables with a 95% confidence interval (CI). A p value < 0.05 was considered as statistically significant.

3. Results

A total of 31 patients were enrolled and randomized to this trial: 15 to the problematic group (with MUF) and 16 to the control group (without MUF).

3.1. Preoperative characteristics

Table 1 shows the type of congenital disease that was operated by means of CPB in both groups of study. There are no differences in the total number of congenital heart disease in the studied groups, but control group (without MUF) showed more patients with AV channel than the problematic group (with MUF).

Congenital heart disease type	Total series (n = 31) n (%)	Problematic group (With MUF) (n = 15) n (%)	Control group (Without MUF) (n = 16) n (%)	P OR (95% CI)
Ventricular septal defect	13 (42%)	8 (52%)	5 (31%)	NS
Balanced AV channel	8 (26%)	1 (7%)	7 (44%)	0.0373 0.09 (0.0096 – 0.8770)
Congenital mitral valve disease	4 (13%)	3 (20%)	1 (6%)	NS
Sub aortic membrane	3 (10%)	1 (7%)	2 (13%)	NS
Right ventricular outflow tract obstruction	1 (3%)	1 (7%)	0 (0%)	NS
Double chamber right ventricle	1 (3%)	1 (7%)	0 (0%)	NS
Atrial septal defect	1 (3%)	0 (0%)	1 (6%)	NS
TOTAL	31 (100%)	15 (100%)	16 (100%)	NS

Table 1. Congenital heart disease type in the studied groups.

Variable	Total series n (%) or mean ± SD (range)	Problematic group (with MUF) n (%) or mean ± SD (range)	Control group (without MUF) n (%) or mean ± SD (range)	p
Age (years)	4.26 ± 4.11 (0.38–17.18)	37 ± 14 (18–76)	31 ± 11 (18–56)	NS
Gender				
Male	12 (39%)	8 (53%)	4 (25%)	NS
Female	19 (61%)	7 (47%)	12 (75%)	NS
Anthropometric data				
Weight (kg)	14.9 ± 10.8 (4–47)	14.1 ± 10.4 (4–38.3)	15.9 ± 11.6 (5.3–47)	NS
Height (cm)	90 ± 31.1 (12–159)	94.2 ± 31.2 (55–158)	86 ± 31.5 (12–159)	NS
Body surface area (m²)	0.56 ± 0.27 (0.25–1.32)	0.58 ± 0.31 (0.25–1.32)	0.53 ± 0.18 (0.28–0.78)	NS
Circulating blood volume (ml)	1032 ± 627 (343–2660)	1164 ± 756 (343–2660)	867 ± 385 (452–1560)	NS
Cardiovascular background				
Previous surgery	0 (0%)	0 (0%)	0 (0%)	NS
Previous catheterization	2 (6%)	0 (0%)	2 (6%)	NS
Pathologic background				
Pre-operative infection	1 (3%)	0 (0%)	1 (6%)	NS
Pulmonary artery hypertension	4 (13%)	0 (0%)	4 (25%)	NS
None	26 (84%)	15 (100%)	11 (69%)	NS
Syndromes				
Down's syndrome	3 (10%)	0 (0%)	3 (19%)	NS
None	28 (90%)	15 (100%)	13 (81%)	NS
NYHA/Ross pre-operative functional class				
I	8 (26%)	4 (27%)	4 (25%)	NS
II	21 (68%)	9 (60%)	12 (75%)	NS
III	2 (6%)	2 (13%)	0 (0%)	NS
Operative risk				
RACHS-1 score	2.4 ± 0.5 (1–3)	2.4 ± 0.5 (2–3)	2.4 ± 0.6 (1–3)	NS
Basic Aristoteles	7.2 ± 1.5 (3–9)	7 ± 1.2 (6–9)	7.4 ± 1.9 (3–9)	NS
Complete Aristoteles	8.1 ± 1.8 (4–11)	7.8 ± 1.5 (6–10)	8.4 ± 2.1 (4–11)	NS
Preoperative morbidity				
Mechanic ventilation	0 (0%)	0 (0%)	0 (0%)	NS
Pre-operative inotropic support	0 (0%)	0 (0%)	0 (0%)	NS
Pre-operative infection	1 (3%)	0 (0%)	1(6%)	NS
None	30 (97%)	15 (100%)	15 (94%)	NS
Pre-operative laboratory exams				
Lactate	1.2 ± 0.3 (0.6–1.7)	1.2 ± 0.3 (0.7–1.7)	1.1 ± 0.3 (0.6–1.5)	NS

Variable	Total series	Problematic group (with MUF)	Control group (without MUF)	p
	n (%) or mean ± SD (range)	n (%) or mean ± SD (range)	n (%) or mean ± SD (range)	
Creatinine	0.4 ± 0.1 (0.2–0.7)	0.4 ± 0.1 (0.2–0.7)	0.4 ± 0.1 (0.3–0.5)	NS
Perfusion variables				
Oxygenator type				
Baby Rx	14 (52%)	7 (47%)	7 (58%)	NS
Terumo SX10	6 (22%)	4 (27%)	2 (17%)	NS
Terumo SX18	1 (4%)	1 (7%)	0 (0%)	NS
Mini max	5 (19%)	2 (13%)	3 (25%)	NS
Safe Mini	1 (4%)	1 (7%)	0 (0%)	NS
Arterial filter use	18 (67%)	12 (80%)	6 (50%)	NS
Surgical variables				
CPB time (min)	81.9 ± 26.9 (40–131)	76.5 ± 23.7 (40–122)	87 ± 29.4 (41–131)	NS
Aortic cross clamp time (min)	53.7 ± 23.6 (12–96)	49.5 ± 21.8 (18–90)	57.6 ± 25.2 (12–96)	NS
Temperature (°C)	27 ± 1.6 (24–30)	27 ± 1.5 (24–29)	27.3 ± 1.8 (24–30)	NS
Anterograde cardioplegia	29 (94%)	14 (93%)	15 (94%)	NS
Blood cardioplegia	29 (94%)	14 (93%)	15 (94%)	NS

Table 2. Pre-operative characteristics of the studied groups.

Table 2 shows the rest of preoperative characteristics in both studied groups. Note that there are no statistical differences in all variables analyzed between the two groups.

Although more random patients with AV channel in the control group, the rest of the preoperative data showed that both groups are absolutely comparable.

3.2. Biochemical operative results

Table 3 compares the concentration of pro-inflammatory agents between groups before surgical correction (T0). Note a baseline elevated concentration of IL-6 in the problematic group (with MUF), without differences in both groups for the rest of pro-inflammatory agents (IL-10, C3d, and C4d).

On the other hand, **Table 4** shows a lack of statistical significant difference in the concentrations of pro-inflammatory agents at the control group before surgical correction (T0) and after CPB (T2).

Finally, **Table 5** shows the comparison between concentration of pro-inflammatory agents in the problematic group before surgical correction (T0) and after MUF (T4). There is a statistically significant removal of IL-6, but no difference in the concentrations of the rest pro-inflammatory agents analyzed (IL-10, C3d, and C4d).

Pro-inflammatory agent	T0 problematic group (with MUF) n = 15 Mean ± DE	T0 control group (without MUF) n = 16 Mean ± DE	p
C3d (ng/ml)	368.66 ± 331.87	413.248 ± 316.804	NS
C4d (ng/ml)	199.57 ± 201.56	213.89 ± 116.72	NS
IL-6 (pg/ml)	**672.249 ± 433.186**	**246.874 ± 365.69**	**0.0061**
IL-10 (pg/ml)	239.698 ± 381.517	299.618 ± 370.148	NS

Table 3. Comparison between concentrations of pro-inflammatory agents in both groups of study (with and without MUF) at baseline (T0).

Pro-inflammatory agent	T0 control group (without MUF) n = 16 Mean ± SD	T2 control group (without MUF) n = 16 Mean ± SD	p
C3d (ng/ml)	413.248 ± 316.804	264.33 ± 198.12	NS
C4d (ng/ml)	213.89 ± 116.72	210.65 ± 141.13	NS
IL-6 (pg/ml)	246.874 ± 365.69	289.499 ± 301.913	NS
IL-10 (pg/ml)	299.618 ± 370.148	387.26 ± 306.07	NS

Table 4. Comparison between concentrations of pro-inflammatory agents at T0 (baseline) and T2 (after CPB) for the control group (without MUF).

3.3. Clinical operative results

Table 6 summarizes the comparison of clinical end point variables in both groups of study (with and without MUF). There is a statistically significant decrease of hemoglobin (Hb) in the problematic group after MUF compared with the baseline level, which is not observed in the control group.

Both groups show an increase in lactate levels and heart rate after surgery when comparing these values with the baseline ones before CPB. Control group (without MUF) showed a

Pro-inflammatory agent	T0 problematic group (with MUF) n = 15 Mean ± SD	T4 problematic group (without MUF) n = 15 Mean ± SD	p
C3d (ng/ml)	368.66 ± 331.87	379.99 ± 264.64	NS
C4d (ng/ml)	199.57 ± 201.56	172.89 ± 139.64	NS
IL-6 (pg/ml)	**672.249 ± 433.186**	**366.31 ± 280.25**	**0.0293**
IL-10 (pg/ml)	239.698 ± 381.517	230.453 ± 352.27	NS

Table 5. Comparison between concentrations of pro-inflammatory agents at baseline (T0) and after MUF (T4) for the problematic group (with MUF).

Operative clinical end point variable	Problematic group (with MUF)			Control group (without MUF)			Problem vs control groups (with vs without MUF)		
	Control group	Problematic group	p	Control group	Problematic group	p	Problematic group	Control group	p
	Before CPB	After MUF		Before CPB	After MUF		After MUF	After CPB	
	n/total n (%) or	n/total n (%) or		n/total n (%) or	n/total n (%) or		n/total n (%) or	n/total n (%) or	
	Mean ± SD	Mean ± SD		Mean ± SD	Mean ± SD		Mean ± SD	Mean ± SD	
Laboratory exams									
Hematocrit (%)	38 ± 7	34 ± 6	NS	37 ± 5	34 ± 7	NS	34 ± 6	34 ± 7	NS
Hemoglobin (g/dl)	14 ± 5	11 ± 2	0.0344	12 ± 2	11 ± 2	NS	11 ± 2	11 ± 2	NS
CPB hematocrit (%)							26 ± 5*	24 ± 4*	NS
Lactate (mmol/L)	1.2 ± 0.3	3.5 ± 1.4	0.0001	1.1 ± 0.3	3.3 ± 1.2	0.0001	3.5 ± 1.4	3.3 ± 1.2	NS
Hemodynamic variables									
Heart rate (beats per minute)	97 ± 15	113 ± 18	0.012	97 ± 16	112 ± 15	0.0116	113 ± 18	112 ± 15	NS
Systolic blood pressure (mmHg)	85 ± 16	89 ± 12	NS	83 ± 10	90 ± 20	NS	89 ± 12	90 ± 20	NS
Diastolic blood pressure (mmHg)	53 ± 15	52 ± 12	NS	49 ± 7	49 ± 12	NS	52 ± 12	49 ± 12	NS
Mean blood pressure (mmHg)	64 ± 18	61 ± 12	NS	64 ± 13	64 ± 17	NS	61 ± 12	64 ± 17	NS
Central venous pressure (mmHg)	10 ± 8	12 ± 7	NS	8 ± 1	10 ± 3	0.0203	12 ± 7	10 ± 3	NS
Operative morbidity and mortality									
Morbidity						3 (20%)	1 (6%)		NS
Mortality						0 (0%)	0 (0%)	0 (0%)	NS

*CPB measured values (due to hemodilution).

Table 6. Comparison between operative clinical end point variables in both groups of study (with and without MUF).

statistically significant increase in central venous pressure after CPB compared with the ones before CPB. There were no differences before and after CPB in the other hemodynamic variables (systolic, diastolic, and mean blood pressures), nor inoperative morbidity and mortality. Successful clinical operative endpoints were archived in both groups of study.

4. Discussion

Cardiopulmonary bypass (CPB) is able to trigger a systemic inflammatory response syndrome (SRIS) due to several factors that include: (1) cell activation secondary to contact with CPB synthetic surfaces, (2) mechanic stress, (3) tissue ischemia and reperfusion, (4) hypotension, (5) non-pulsatile flow, (6) hemodilution relative anemia, (7) blood and blood products transfusion, (8) heparin and protamine administration, and (9) hypothermic effects. CPB activates the vessels endothelium and releases pro-inflammatory agents such as tumoral necrosis factor α (TNF-α), interleukins, and endotoxins. These agents also activate the intracellular transcription factor that increases endothelial pro-inflammatory cytokines and the molecular expression of leukocyte adhesion.

It is well known the fact that younger age increases even more the inflammatory effects of CPB. Some reasons include increased metabolic demand in these patients, hyperactivity of their pulmonary vessels, immaturity of their organs/systems, and altered homeostasis. The risk is particularly high in neonates and young infants due to mismatch between CPB and patient's size, with CPB circuit volume usually 200–300% higher than that of the patient. Additionally, an increased metabolic demand requires elevated pump flow up to 200 ml/kg^{-1}/min^{-1} in neonates. Combining a relative major size of CPB with an increased perfusion rate leads to a greater blood exposure to synthetic surfaces of the circuit components [23]. In our series, there was no age difference between the studied groups, and it is important to highlight that none of the groups included neonate patients for the reasons already discussed.

One of the most involved cytokines in SRIS development is, indeed, IL-6. Increased concentrations of IL-6 have been reported in patients with postoperative complications, and a correlation with posterior left ventricular wall dyskinesia detected by means of transesophageal echocardiography has been established. IL-6 is also an endogenous pyrogen agent that activates acute phase reactant proteins. Concentration of IL-6 increases independently of the oxygenator type, degree of hypothermia, or heparin use in the CPB circuit surfaces [24, 25]. Although in our study IL-6 concentrations were significantly higher before surgery in the problematic group than in the control group, this agent is also the one that is significantly more removed by MUF. This is probably the most relevant fact of our study because it shows that the benefit of MUF in congenital heart disease surgery is the removal of IL-6, an important pro-inflammatory agent, particularly in patients that SRIS is enhanced because of the immaturity of their immune system. Another effect that is important to discuss is the fact that, if MUF benefits patients with simple congenital heart disease surgery as were the ones included in our study, it would indeed improve operative outcomes in those operated on for complex congenital heart disease [26]. This single fact justifies the routine use of MUF in all patients with congenital heart disease that is operated on with CPB.

There are several additional methods, despite ultrafiltration, that had been developed in order to diminish SRIS secondary to CPB at surgical correction of congenital heart disease in pediatric population. Some of them are steroids (e.g., dexamethasone 10–30 mg/kg 6–12 hours before CPB) and modified tubular synthetic surfaces in the CPB circuit. However, none of these methods is as such as useful for this purpose as MUF, which is established right after ending the CPB and before decannulation of the patient [27]. Since 1973, different types of hemofilters have been developed in order to remove priming volume (water) following the principle of pressure gradient, particularly those made of polycarbonate. These filters have been replaced by the ones made out of polysulfonate in 1986 and later by the current generation of polyamide hemofilters. These are the most practical ones because of its greater biocompatibility, reduced surface, and more ultrafiltration effectiveness due to a less than physiological pressure.

The effectiveness of ultrafiltration for removing pro-inflammatory agents depends also on the type of hemofilter and on the modality of ultrafiltration procedure used. Kosik et al comments Berdat´s study on the effectiveness of polysulfonate filters vs polyamide ones in the two ultrafiltration modalities for the removal of pro-inflammatory agents such as IL-6, IL-10, and TNFα [3]. They prove that IL-6 was better removed by conventional ultrafiltration (CUF) with poliariletersulfonate filter, while TNFα was better removed by modified ultrafiltration (MUF) and poliariletersulfonate filter. The rest of the pro-inflammatory agents was not modified neither for the ultrafiltration modality nor for the hemofilter type. Therefore, it seems that MUF with poliariletersulfonate hemofilter is the better strategy for removing pro-inflammatory agents in pediatric patients with congenital heart surgery. Our results are based on the ultrafiltration modality rather than the type of filter, since the material of hemofilters that we used was variable.

It has been reported that MUF is not only useful for removing extracellular fluid excess, but also cytokines and other inflammatory agents triggered by CPB and surgical trauma. There is some controversy in the literature regarding the efficacy of filters in the removal of cytokines, as well as in the differences between the two ultrafiltration modalities [28]. Additionally, the comparative results between both ultrafiltration modalities are difficult to interpret due to variations in the ultrafiltration technique, equipment, definitions and objectives, and measurements of cytokines. Finally, it is still not known if the clinical benefits of MUF are due to the removal of cytokines and other inflammatory agents, or to the isolated reduction of tissue edema [29–33].

5. Conclusion

Based on the results of this study [34], we can say that although the baseline concentrations of IL-6 in the patients of the problematic group were higher in relation to those of the control group, the removal of this pro-inflammatory agent by MUF was statistically significant. This indicates that MUF is a procedure that can benefit pediatric patients with congenital heart disease undergoing CPB because it is able to decrease the concentration of IL-6. Therefore, we consider that the use of MUF in pediatric patients should be routinely recommended as long as hemodynamic conditions allow it.

Acknowledgements

We thank the Cardio Slim Foundation for the financial support provided to carry out this study.

Conflict of interest

The authors declare no potential conflicts of interest with respect to the research, authorship or publication of this manuscript.

Author details

Pedro José Curi-Curi[1]*, Elizabeth Aguilar Alanis[1], Juan Calderón-Colmenero[2],
Jorge Luis Cervantes-Salazar[1], Rodrigo Reyes Pavón[1] and Samuel Ramírez-Marroquín[1]

*Address all correspondence to: pcuricuri001@gmail.com

1 Department of Congenital Heart Disease and Pediatric Cardiac Surgery, "Ignacio Chávez" National Cardiology Institute, Mexico City, Mexico

2 Department of Pediatric Cardiology, "Ignacio Chávez" National Cardiology Institute, Mexico City, Mexico

References

[1] Brix-Christensen V. The systemic inflammatory response after cardiac surgery with cardiopulmonary bypass in children. Acta Anaesthesiologica Scandinavica. 2001;45:671-679

[2] Seghaye MC. The clinical implications of the systemic inflammatory reaction related to cardiac operations in children. Cardiology in the Young. 2003;13:228-239

[3] Kozik D, Tweddell J. Characterizing the inflammatory response to cardiopulmonary bypass in children. The Annals of Thoracic Surgery. 2006;81:S2347-S2354

[4] Kirklin JK, Westaby S, Blackstone EH, Kirklin JW, Chenowelh DE, Pacifico AD. Complement and the damaging effects of cardiopulmonary bypass. Journal of Thoracic and Cardiovascular Surgery. 1983;86:845-847

[5] Seghaye M, Duchateau J, Grabitz RG, Nitsch G, Marcus C, Messmer BJ, von Bernuth G. Complement, leukocytes and leukocyte elastase in full-term neonates undergoing cardiac operation. Journal of Thoracic and Cardiovascular Surgery. 1994;108:29-36

[6] Seghaye M, Grabitz RG, Duchateau J, Bussea S, Däbritz S, Koch D, et al. Inflammatory reaction and capillary leak syndrome related to cardiopulmonary bypass in neonates undergoing cardiac operations. Journal of Thoracic and Cardiovascular Surgery. 1996; **112**:687-697

[7] Ashraf SS, Tian Y, Zacharrias S, Cowan D, Martin P, Watterson K. Effects of cardiopulmonary bypass on neonatal and paediatric inflammatory profiles. European Journal of Cardio-Thoracic Surgery. 1997;**12**:862-868

[8] McBride WT, McBride SJ. The balance of pro- and anti-inflammatory cytokines in cardiac surgery. Current Opinion in Anesthesiology. 1998;**11**:15-22

[9] McBride WT, Armstrong MA, Gilliland H, McMurray TJ. The balance of pro- and anti-inflammatory cytokines in plasma and bronchoalveolar lavage (BAL) at paediatric cardiac surgery. Cytokine. 1996;**8**:724-729

[10] Chevv M, Brandslund I, Brix-Christensen V, et al. Tissue injury and the inflammatory response to pediatric cardiac surgery with cardiopulmonary bypass. Anesthesiology. 2001;**94**:745-753

[11] Finn A, Moat N, Rebuck N, Klein N, Slrobel S, Elliott M. Changes in neutrophil CDllb/CD18 and L-selectin expression and release of interleukin 8 and elastase in paediatric cardiopulmonay bypass. Agents and Actions. 1993;**38**:C44-C46

[12] Brix-Christensen V, Petersen TK, Ravn HB, Hjortdal VE, Andersen NR, Tonnesen E. Cardiopulmonary bypass elicits a pro- and anti-inflammatory response and impaired chemotaxis in neonatal pigs. Acta Anaesthesiologica Scandinavica. 2001;**45**:407-413

[13] Hennein HA, Kiseltepe U, Barst S, Bocchieri KA, Remick DG, et al. Venovenous modified ultrafiltration after cardiopulmonary bypass in children: A prospective randomized study. Journal of Thoracic and Cardiovascular Surgery. 1999;**117**:496-505

[14] Kern FH, Morana NJ, Sears JJ, Hickey PR. Coagulation defects in neonates during cardiopulmonary bypass. The Annals of Thoracic Surgery. 1992;**54**:541-546

[15] Boga M, Islamoglu F, Badak I, Cikirikcioglu M, Bakalim T, Yagdi T. The effects of modified hemofiltration on inflammatory mediators and cardiac performance in coronary artery bypass grafting. Perfusion. 2000;**15**:143-150

[16] Tassani P, Richter JA, Eising GP, Barabkay A, Braun SL, Haehnel CH, et al. Influence of combined zero-balanced and modified ultrafiltration on the systemic inflammatory response during coronary artery bypass grafting. Journal of Cardiothoracic and Vascular Anesthesia. 1999;**13**:285-291

[17] Pearl JM, Manning PB, McNamara JL, Saucier MM, Thomas DW. Effect of modified ultrafiltration on plasma thromboxane B2, leukotriene B4, endothelin-1 in infants undergoing cardiopulmonary bypass. The Annals of Thoracic Surgery. 1999;**68**:1369-1375

[18] Grunenfelder J, Sund G, Schoeberlein A, Maly FE, Guntli S, Fischer K, et al. Modified ultrafiltration lowers adhesion molecule and cytokine levels after cardiopulmonary bypass without clinical relevance in adults. European Journal of Cardio-Thoracic Surgery. 2000;**17**:77-83

[19] Chew MS. Does modified ultrafiltration reduce the systemic inflammatory response to cardiac surgery with cardiopulmonary bypass? Perfusion. 2004;**19**:S57-S60

[20] Hauser GJ, Ben-Ari J, Colvin MP, Dalton HJ, Hertzog JH, Bearb M, et al. Interleukin-6 levels in serum and lung lavage fluid of children undergoing open heart surgery correlate with postoperative morbidity. Intensive Care Medicine. 1998;**24**:481-486

[21] Gilliland HE, Armstrong MA, McMurray TJ. The inflammatory response to pediatric cardiac surgery: Correlation of granulocyte adhesion molecule expression with postoperative oxygenation. Anesthesia & Analgesia. 1999;**89**:1188-1191

[22] Andreasson S, Góthberg S, Berggren H, Bengtsson A, Eriksson E, Risberg B. Hemofiltration modifies complement activation after extracorporeal circulation in infants. The Annals of Thoracic Surgery. 1993;**56**:1515-1517

[23] Wang W, Chiu I, Chao-Min W, Pei-Lin L, Huand HM, Chung-I C, et al. Modified ultrafiltration in pediatric cardiopulmonary bypass. Perfusion. 1998;**13**:304-310

[24] Ming-Jiuh W, Chiu I-S, Chao-Ming W, Pei-Lin L, Chung-I C, Chi-Hsiang H, Shu-Hsun C. Efficacy of ultrafiltration in removing inflammatory mediators during pediatric cardiac operations. The Annals of Thoracic Surgery. 1996;**61**:651-656

[25] Naik S, Knight A, Elliott MJ. A prospective randomized study of a modified technique of ultrafiltration during pediatric open-heart surgery. Circulation. 1991;**84**(Suppl III): 422-431

[26] Bando K, Turrentine MW, Vijay P, Sharp TG, Lalone BJ, et al. Effect of modified ultrafiltration in high-risk patients undergoing operations for congenital heart disease. The Annals of Thoracic Surgery. 1998;**66**:821-828

[27] Draasima AM, Hazekamp MG, Frank M, Anes N, Schoof PH, Huysmans HA. Modified ultrafiltration after cardiopulmonary bypass in pediatric cardiac surgery. The Annals of Thoracic Surgery. 1997;**64**:521-525

[28] Daggett CW, Lodge AJ, Scarborough JE, Chai PJ, Jaggers J, Ungerleider RM. Modified ultrafiltration versus conventional ultrafiltration: A randomized prospective study in neonatal piglets. Journal of Thoracic and Cardiovascular Surgery. 1998;**H5**:336-342

[29] Davies MJ, Nguyen K, Gaynor JW, Elliott MJ. Modified ultrafiltration improves left ventricular systolic function in infants after cardiopulmonary bypass. Journal of Thoracic and Cardiovascular Surgery. 1998;**5**:361-370

[30] Journois D, Israel-Biet D, Pouard P, Rolland B, Silvester W, Vouhe P, Safran D, et al. High-volume, zero-balanced hemofiltration to reduce delayed inflammatory response to cardiopulmonary bypass in children. Anesthesiology. 1996;**85**:965-976

[31] Chew MS, Brix-Christensen V, Ravn H, Brandslund I, Ditlevsen E, Pedersen J, et al. Effect of modified ultrafiltration on the inflammatory response in paediatric open-heart surgery: A prospective, randomized study. Perfusion. 2002;**17**:327-333

[32] Ramamoorthy C, Lynn AM. The use of modified ultrafiltration during pediatric cardiovascular surgery is not a benefit. Journal of Cardiothoracic and Vascular Anesthesia. 1998;**12**(4):483-485

[33] García-Montes JA, Calderón-Colmenero J, Juanico A. Cuidados Intensivos en el niño cardiópata. In: Attie F, Calderón-Colmenero J, Zabal C, Buendía A, editors. Cardiología Pediátrica. México DF: Editorial Médica Panamericana; 2013. p. 203

[34] Curi-Curi PJ, del Villar MRS, Gómez-García L, Vergara BG, Calderón-Colmenero J, Ramírez-Marroquín S, Cervantes-Salazar JL. Impacto intraoperatorio de la ultrafil-tración modificada en pacientes pediátricos sometidos a cirugía cardíaca con circulación extracorpórea. Cirugía Cardiovascular. 2016;**23**(4):179-186

Chapter 5

The Adult with Coarctation of the Aorta

Ayesha Salahuddin, Alice Chan and Ali N. Zaidi

Additional information is available at the end of the chapter

http://dx.doi.org/10.5772/intechopen.79865

Abstract

The manuscript will discuss the epidemiology and etiology of the adult with coarctation of the aorta (CoA) as well as describe the embryology, anatomy, pathophysiology, and clinical presentation in order to recognize and appropriately diagnose an adult patient with CoA. This chapter will also review diagnostic testing, management, therapeutic interventions including percutaneous and surgical procedures, and long-term complications that can arise in an adult with repaired CoA. It contains images with examples from echocardiography, cardiac computed tomography (CT), magnetic resonance imaging (MRI), and angiograms as part of the description.

Keywords: congenital heart disease, coarctation of the aorta, percutaneous intervention, balloon dilatation, stenting, surgery, management, complications

1. Introduction

Coarctation of the aorta is a congenital cardiac defect. It usually manifests as a discrete constriction of the aortic isthmus. However, it is more likely to represent a spectrum of aortic narrowing from this discrete entity to tubular hypoplasia, with many variations seen in between these two extremes. Morphologists argue that tubular hypoplasia, although it may coexist with discrete coarctation, should be considered as a separate entity [1]. On rare occasions there can be a gap between the ascending and descending thoracic aorta, known as an interrupted aortic arch. Interventions can be required as an infant however procedures may be needed later in life for native coarctation or patients with recurrent coarctation. The presence of associated arch hypoplasia is relevant to longer term risk for the development of hypertension so in addition to re-coarctation, these patients are at increased risk for developing other comorbidities and should have lifelong follow up care.

2. Epidemiology

Coarctation of the aorta (CoA) is the fifth most common congenital heart defect, accounting for 6–8% of live births with congenital heart disease, with an estimated incidence of 1 in 2500 births [2–5]. It affects more male babies than female, with a reported ratio in males of between 1.27:1 and 1.74:1 [6, 7]. Patients with CoA can have other defects like atrial septal defect (ASD), ventricular septal defect (VSD), atrioventricular canal defect (AVCD), bicuspid aortic valve (BAV), transposition of great arteries (TGA), patent ductus arteriosus (PDA), hypoplastic left heart syndrome. CoA often coexists with other left heart obstructive lesions like mitral stenosis, subaortic stenosis and aortic stenosis. About 50–60% patients with coarctation of the aorta or interrupted aortic arch have a BAV [8]. Compared to right-sided lesions, left-sided cardiac obstructions are more frequently seen in males than female [2]. One genetic condition noted to be associated with an increased risk of having coarctation of the aorta (12–35%) is Turner syndrome [9]. Lastly, the etiology of CoA is not well understood and thought to be affected by various factors including a genetic component, environmental factors, and arteriopathy.

3. Etiology and cardiac associations

The etiology of the discrete isthmic constriction of the aorta seen in patients with CoA remains controversial and is thought to be multifactorial. Although the precise pathogenesis is unknown, the two theories for the development of congenital coarctation of the aorta have been postulated: reduced antegrade intrauterine blood flow causing underdevelopment of the fetal aortic arch [10] and migration or extension of ductal tissue into the wall of the fetal thoracic aorta [11]. Histologic examination of localized aortic coarctation lesions has demonstrated the presence of a tissue ridge extending from the posterior aortic wall and protruding into aortic lumen. This ridge consists of ductal tissue with in-folding of the aortic media [12]. Prenatal environmental exposures have been associated with CoA and other left-sided lesions. However, there is a growing body of literature that suggests a genetic basis for development of these lesions [13]. There has been evidence of genetic contribution to CoA [14, 15]. Vascular endothelial growth factor (VEGF) plays a vital role in aortic development, acting as a chemo-attractant, stimulating angioblast migration toward the midline before formation of the aorta. Indeed, targeted disruption of VEGF in mice leads to significant disruption of the developing aorta [16]. Whether an initial mutation leads to secondary effects on VEGF or on other signaling systems involved in recruiting mural cells in fetuses, leading to CoA, is unknown. An increase in collagen and decrease in smooth muscle content of the pre-coarctation aorta in humans has been demonstrated in comparison to post-coarctation aorta or to proximal aorta of young transplant donors [17]. Recently, mutations in the NOTCH1 gene have been identified in individuals with left ventricular outflow tract malformation, including coarctation [18]. Up to 18–30% of patients with Turner syndrome have coarctation [19]. Genetic testing for Turner syndrome (i.e., karyotype analysis) should therefore be performed in female patients diagnosed with coarctation of the aorta [20, 21]. Mechanical models have suggested that abnormalities of blood flow, defective endothelial cell migration, and excessive deposition of aortic duct tissue at the aortic isthmus can result in coarctation [22]. Epidemiological studies have found that for left ventricular outflow tract lesions, there is a higher chance of concordant diagnosis in multiple family members [23]. The co-existence of CoA with other left heart obstructive pathologies like aortic stenosis and hypoplastic left heart syndrome suggests that there could be a common pathogenic mechanism at a molecular level [24, 25]. Williams syndrome, a congenital and multisystem genetic disorder, has been associated with supravalvular aortic stenosis. Aortic arch abnormalities, including coarctation, are present in 10% of patients with Williams syndrome [26]. Coarctation can also be present in congenital cardiovascular anomalies involving multiple left-sided lesions, including Shone syndrome and hypoplastic left heart syndrome [22]. Environmental factors could also play a role in the incidence of CoA since there is increase CoA rate along the US-Mexico border [27]. Seasonal variations have been reported in the incidence of CoA we well [28].

4. Noncardiac associations

The link between intracranial aneurysms and CoA was described well before the surgical era, accounting for 5% deaths in patients with aortic coarctation on autopsy review [29]. Most of the aneurysms described are small, and therefore have a low risk of spontaneous rupture. Currently the benefits of routine screening for intracranial aneurysms in coarctation remain unclear [22].

5. Anatomy

Although most patients have a discrete narrowing of the descending aorta at the insertion of the ductus arteriosus, there is a spectrum of aortic narrowing that encompasses the usual discrete thoracic lesions, long-segmental defects, tubular hypoplasia, and, rarely, coarctation located in the abdominal aorta. In simple terms, coarctation is characterized by discrete narrowing of the thoracic aorta adjacent to the ligamentum arteriosum. Importantly, discrete coarctation is an aortopathy that lies within a spectrum of arch abnormalities ranging from discrete narrowing to a long segment of arch hypoplasia. Morphologically it appears as a localized shelf in the posterolateral aortic wall. There are some anatomic variations of coarctation. It maybe appear as (a) discrete narrowing (b) tubular hypoplasia of any part of the arch or (c) aortic arch interruption [30]. CoA has also been described as a diffuse arteriopathy with abnormalities in the elastic properties of the aorta. Increase in collagen and decreases in smooth muscle component of the pre-coarctation aorta have been reported [31].

Although CoA can be an isolated CHD, it is also commonly found in other congenital syndromes and cardiovascular anomalies. Thus, deliberate investigation for the presence of coarctation should be made in these patients. The most common cardiovascular malformation associated with CoA is BAV. Prior autopsy examination showed 46% of patients with CoA have congenital BAV [32]. The relative frequency of associated cardiac lesions in patients with CoA differs somewhat based upon the age of the population studies. Adult patients with CoA evaluated with magnetic resonance imaging, 17% had no additional cardiovascular anomalies however, in this cohort, BAV, arch hypoplasia, VSD, and PDA were detected in 60, 14, 13, and 7% of patients, respectively [33]. The coincidence of BAV and CoA is difficult to determine, because BAV is very common and not everyone is screened for the presence of coarctation.

6. Pathophysiology and presentation

The clinical presentation of coarctation differs significantly in pediatric patients in comparison with adults. Although infants with severe coarctation may present with signs and symptoms of heart failure and cardiogenic shock as the ductus closes, most adults with unrepaired coarctation are generally asymptomatic. A common presentation of coarctation is systemic arterial hypertension. The causes of hypertension in this cohort of patients are not fully understood, but malfunction in a number of individual systems have been implicated, including imbalance within the autonomic nervous system [34], impaired vascular function [35, 36] and hyperactivation of the rennin–angiotensin system [37, 38]. It is likely that more than one of these systems is involved. In young adults presenting with severe upper extremity hypertension, coarctation should be excluded. Patients presenting with severe hypertension may experience symptoms including angina, headache, epistaxis, and heart failure [22]. Coarctation causes upper extremity hypertension, which leads to systemic hypertension and left ventricular hypertrophy. There have been several mechanisms proposed for hypertension in patients with coarctation, which include reduced arterial compliance, blunted baroreceptor sensitivity and endothelial dysfunction [39]. Age at repair is an important determinant of developing late hypertension. Patients who get the repair in infancy have less than 5% chance of developing hypertension by early adulthood, whereas those operated on after the age of one have a 25–33% chance of developing hypertension [40–42]. Late hypertension is associated with residual or recurrent obstruction. Despite the variability in blood pressure in the upper and lower extremities, regional blood flow is generally maintained within normal limits by autoregulatory vasoconstriction in the hypertensive areas and by vasodilation in the hypotensive areas [43]. Nonetheless some patients with satisfactory repair can still develop late hypertension due to vascular dysfunction [44]. In a systemic review of literature, the median prevalence of late hypertension after satisfactory repair was reported to be 32% with a range of 25–68% [45]. Ambulatory blood pressure monitoring can help in early diagnosis of late hypertension [46]. Patients with coarctation remain at a high risk of developing complications like premature coronary atherosclerosis, cerebrovascular events, left ventricular systolic dysfunction and endocarditis. With early repair, timely recognition of late hypertension and treatment of risk factors, the overall survival has improved. However, the life expectancy of these individuals is not as normal as the unaffected peers [47].

In full term newborns one of the important causes of congestive heart failure is aortic coarctation. Beyond the neonatal period most patients are asymptomatic and present with difficult to control hypertension in later years. In previously undiagnosed adults, the classic presenting sign is hypertension. Older patients might complain of headaches, leg fatigue with exercise and cold extremities. As mentioned previously, coarctation can be a part of syndromes like

Turner syndrome, Williams Syndrome or Shone's complex. Almost 50% of the cases are associated with BAV. Other associated abnormalities include intracranial aneurysms (most commonly of the circle of Willis) in 2–10% case and acquired intercostal artery aneurysms [30]. Data on the natural history of coarctation of the aorta are largely derived from hospital post-mortem records and from case series prior to the availability of operative repair that was first done in 1945 [48]. The average survival age of individuals with unoperated coarctation was approximately 35 years of age, with 75% mortality by 46 years of age [49]. Common complications in unoperated patients or in those operated on during later childhood or adulthood were systemic hypertension, accelerated coronary artery disease, stroke, aortic dissection, and heart failure. Causes of death include heart failure, aortic rupture, aortic dissection, endocarditis, endarteritis, intra-cerebral hemorrhage, and myocardial infarction [48, 50]. Patients with an associated BAV may also develop significant aortic stenosis, aortic regurgitation, and dilated ascending aorta from myxomatous degeneration of the medial wall of the aorta.

6.1. Pregnancy and coarctation

Coarctation of the aorta and associated lesions, particularly BAV, aortic stenosis, and ascending aorta dilation should be evaluated before pregnancy for appropriate counseling and advice. Rarely the first manifestation is during pregnancy. In the absence of hemodynamically significant stenotic lesion, pregnancy is well tolerated in patients with repaired aortic coarctation. However there is a greater propensity of developing hypertension during pregnancy [51]. Outcome of pregnancy in patients after repair of aortic coarctation have been reported over the last decade [52]. During pregnancy and delivery, there were no serious cardiovascular complications. Hypertension alone was reported in 21 pregnancies in 14 women, and preeclampsia in 5 pregnancies in 4 women. In another study, serious complications were uncommon in women with a hemodynamically significant gradient ($\geq$20 mmHg) after repair [53]. These women were more likely to have systemic hypertension related to the increased coarctation gradient. However, there are case reports of aortic rupture or dissection that occur with pregnancy after coarctation repair due to the hemodynamic and aortic medial changes of pregnancy, which remain rare.

7. Physical exam

On physical examination, femoral arterial pulses are diminished and usually delayed. Rarely, claudication may be reported because of lower extremity ischemia. Auscultation of the left sternal border may demonstrate a harsh systolic murmur with radiation to the back. An associated thrill may be palpable in the suprasternal notch. If left ventricular pressure or volume overload have developed, a left ventricular lift can be present. The finding of a continuous murmur may suggest the presence of arterial collaterals in those with long-standing unre-paired significant coarctation [22].

If aortic coarctation is suspected blood pressure should be measured in both arms and legs in supine position. Normally BP in the lower extremities is 10–20% higher than the upper extremities due to wave amplification. If BP in the leg is lower than the arm BP by 10 mmHg or more then coarctation should be suspected. A pressure gradient of 35 mmHg or greater is considered highly specific for coarctation [54]. The presence of collateral vessels may diminish the pressure gradient. Arterial pulsations from collaterals to the intercostal and interscapular arteries can also be palpated. In patients with suspected coarctation, it is important to assess for systolic blood pressure discrepancy between upper and lower extremities. The upper extremity systolic blood pressure is usually 20 mmHg higher than the lower extremities in patients with significant coarctation. In rare instances of coarctation patients with concomitant anomalous subclavian artery origin distal to the coarctation, systolic blood pressure differences may not be detected between ipsilateral arm and legs. On auscultation a continuous murmur of aortoaortic collateral arteries would be audible in the interscapular space. Simultaneous palpitation of radial and femoral artery might reveal a delay or absence of the femoral pulse.

8. Diagnostic evaluation

8.1. Initial workup

The electrocardiogram of a patient with coarctation may be normal or demonstrate evidence of left ventricular hypertrophy from chronic left ventricular pressure overload. On chest radiograph, a "figure of three" sign formed by the aortic nob, the stenotic segment, and the dilated post stenotic segment of the aorta suggests CoA. The heart border can be normal or mildly enlarged. Inferior rib notching can also be seen in the third to eighth ribs bilaterally caused by the presence of dilated intercostal collateral arteries [22, 30].

8.2. Echocardiography

Transthoracic echocardiography is the most accessible and the main stay for the practicing physician. A comprehensive echocardiogram is recommended in the initial evaluation of a patient with repaired or suspected CoA. In addition to characterization of the coarctation itself, it is important to evaluate for evidence of left ventricular pressure or volume overload, left ventricular hypertrophy, size, and left ventricular systolic and diastolic dysfunction. Particular attention should be placed in identifying associated cardiac defects especially left-sided lesions. The morphology of the aortic valve, and evidence of subvalvular, valvular, and supravalvular aortic stenosis should be interrogated. The dimensions of the aortic root and ascending aorta can be followed serially to assess for associated aortopathy. Suprasternal windows are important to view the aortic arch from the long-axis view, in two-dimensional imaging and by color flow Doppler. Visualization of the aortic arch in the long axis may demonstrate a focal area of narrowing of the thoracic aorta distal to the takeoff of the left subclavian artery with associated flow turbulence on color flow Doppler.

Coarctation is imaged from the high left parasternal views with lateral angulation of the probe toward the left shoulder. The suprasternal notch view is used for obtaining Doppler gradient (**Figures 1** and **2**). Subcostal imaging is used to evaluate the distal thoracic and upper abdominal aorta. The stenotic segment may be discrete, segmental or long therefore the entire aortic arch should be imaged particularly the origin of the left subclavian artery as in transverse arch hypoplasia the distance between the origin of the left common carotid artery and left subclavian artery may be increased. Low frequency imaging and harmonic imaging can improve the image quality.

On doppler imaging color flow aliasing would be seen at and beyond the narrow segment. Systolic velocity in the descending aorta is increased. If transverse arch hypoplasia is present the proximal velocity increases as well therefore the systolic pressure gradient should be calculated with the expanded Bernoulli equation 4 $(V2^2-V1^2)$ [55, 56]. In severe cases there is a gradient during both systole and diastole across the stenosis, which results in the classic saw tooth pattern. The presence of collateral arteries can cause doppler to underestimate the severity of obstruction [57]. Some of the other factors, which can affect the Doppler gradient, include severe obstruction, long tortuous vessels or eccentric gradient. Yet with long-standing coarctation, significant collaterals may have developed thereby reducing the peak systolic gradient across the site of stenosis. A saw-tooth pattern seen on continuous-wave Doppler reflects the persistent forward flow in diastole because of diastolic run-off. Higher gradient across the coarctation and longer duration of diastolic forward flow in the thoracic aorta suggest more significant coarctation [22].

In the absence of proximal obstruction when the pulse wave doppler is placed in the abdominal aorta, the wave form shows a rapid systolic upstroke, short deceleration time, followed by a brief early diastolic flow reversal and little anterograde flow throughout diastole. In the presence of coarctation there is loss of early diastolic flow reversal, which is highly sensitive

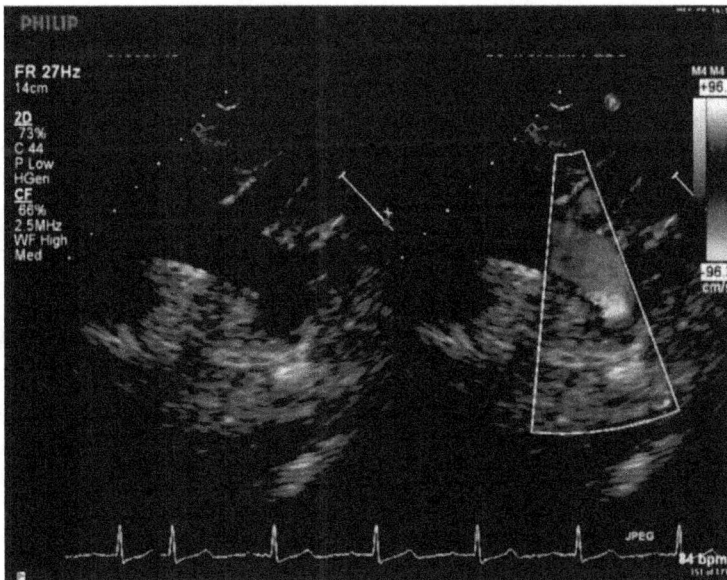

Figure 1. 2D transthoracic echo imaging showing coarctation of the aorta distal to the left subclavian artery.

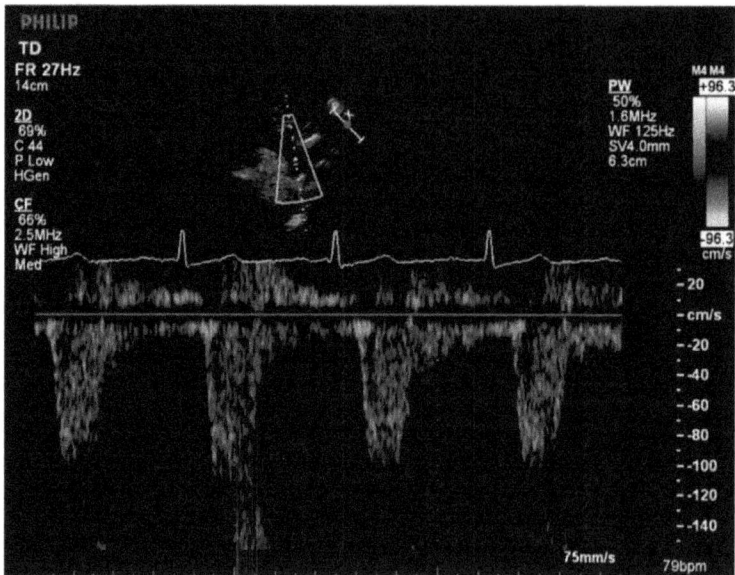

Figure 2. Pulse wave doppler profile through the coarctation segment demonstrating a pressure gradient.

for detection of upstream obstruction. The systolic velocity is blunted, there is continuous anterograde flow and increased diastolic flow velocity. If the delay between R wave on ECG and peak velocity of the abdominal aorta is >50 ms it is associated with coarctation [58].

8.3. Magnetic resonance imaging

Magnetic resonance imaging (MRI) is the most comprehensive method of evaluating coarctation of the aorta. MRI does not expose the patients to ionizing radiations, which is an important consideration for young patients who would have to undergo serial imaging. Cardiac MRI (cMRI) has become a valuable noninvasive modality to assess patients with unrepaired and repaired coarctation. In adults with suboptimal echocardiographic imaging window, cMRI can be used to characterize the aortic valve, aortic root, left ventricular size, and function. cMRI, along with gadolinium-enhanced magnetic resonance angiography, provides excellent resolution of cardiac anatomy and vascular structures. Compared with echocardiography, cMRI demonstrates superior visualization of the aortic arch with precise characterization of the location and extent of coarctation, and assessment of the presence and extent of collateral vessels. n the unrepaired patient, the measured minimum aortic cross-sectional area and heart rate–corrected deceleration time in the descending aorta can be used to predict a significant gradient by cardiac catheterization [59] and future need for interventions. cMRI provides exceptional visualization of the aortic arch and detection of post repair complications including arch "kinking" and pseudoaneurysms. Thoracic aortic magnetic resonance angiography also provides assessment of post stenotic dilation or aneurysmal formation at the site of a previous repair. Importantly, the lack of ionizing radiation provides an advantage of cMRI over CT, in the serial evaluation of late complications after repair [22, 59].

A stack of half-Fourier acquisition single shot turbo spin-echo (HASTE) images of the mediastinum are acquired in transverse, coronal and oblique sagittal plane parallel to the plane of the
aortic arch. These provide dark blood images, which give anatomical overview of the coarctation. Black blood images are less susceptible to artifact from metallic objects. For evaluation
of left ventricular function and mass a stack of steady state free precession (SSFP) cine images
is acquired in the left ventricular short axis plane. Long axis cine images are acquired in the
four, two and three chamber planes. SSFP cine images are then performed through the aortic
root in the plane of the aortic valve, the aortic arch and the region of the aortic isthmus. Phase
contrast flow imaging is performed to quantify the flow volumes and velocity [60].

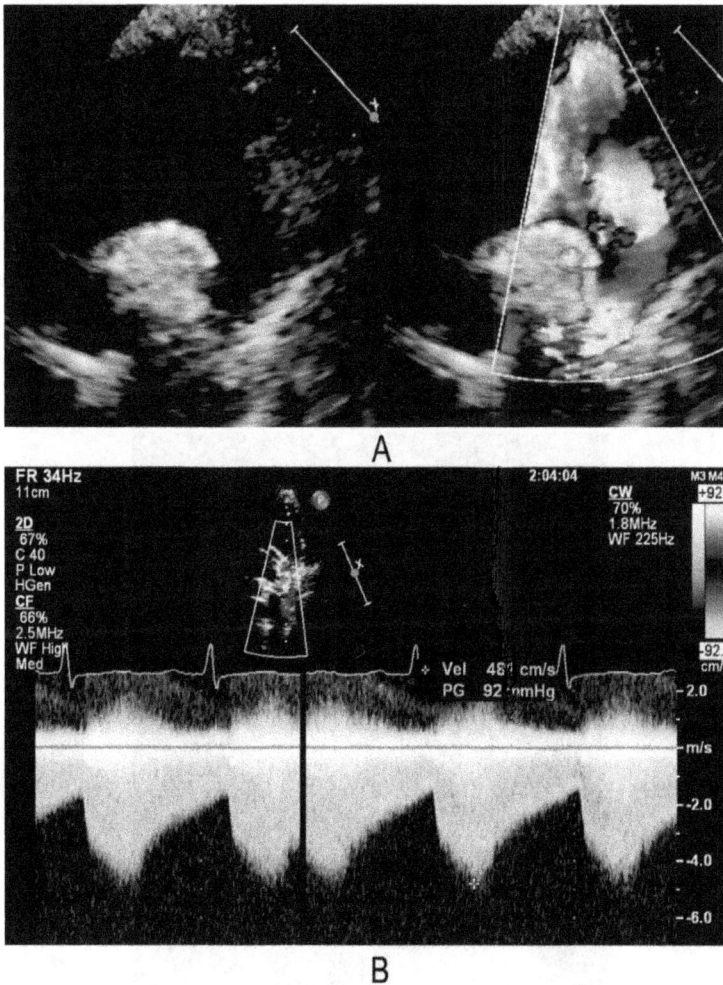

Figure 3. (A) 2D echo with color flow doppler showing severe narrowing of the proximal descending aorta with
significant turbulence and a peak velocity of 4.8 m/s consistent with severe aortic coarctation. (B) Doppler tracing shows
delay in return to baseline in diastole (diastolic drag) and blunting of the abdominal aortic doppler pattern consistent
with significant aortic coarctation.

With phase contrast imaging the degree of collateral flow can be determined. The flow volume is assessed in the aorta just proximal to the stenosis and then at the level of the diaphragm. Usually there is a 7% decrease in total flow from proximal to distal aorta, if there is increase in flow by 5% or more, it is highly indicative of collateral flow joining the descending aorta [61]. Four-dimensional flow MR imaging is an emerging tool to evaluate hemodynamic significance of collateral blood flow (**Figure 3**) [62].

8.4. Computed tomographic angiography (CTA)

Although cMRI is the preferred mode of serial follow-up for patients after coarctation repair, the use of cardiovascular CT may be considered in selected patients. In particular, cMRI in patients with transcatheter stents may have susceptibility artifact precluding accurate assessment of late complications associated with these interventions. With cMRI, metallic artifact can lead to difficulty in the assessment of vessel lumen patency, identifying restenosis, aneurysm, or stent fracture [22]. Use of CT obviates concerns about metallic artifact impairing accurate assessment of stented segments of the aorta. Other advantages of cardiac CT over cMRI include improved image resolution, shorter scan time, and greater availability [22]. CTA is also used to assess concomitant coronary anomalies that may not be well visualized with cMRI. Patients with pacemakers or implantable cardioverter defibrillators that are not cMRI compatible may benefit from surveillance with cardiovascular CTA. Similar to cMRI, cardiovascular CT can be performed to image the coarctation segment, any aneurysmal dilation distal to the coarctation segment, recoarctation post repair, (**Figures 4–7**), hypoplasia of the

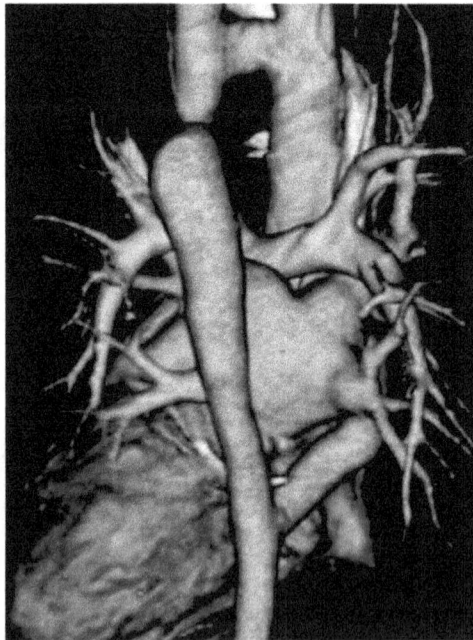

Figure 4. 3D reconstruction (CT angiogram) showing discrete segment of CoA and mild dilatation of the descending thoracic aorta distal to coarctation segment.

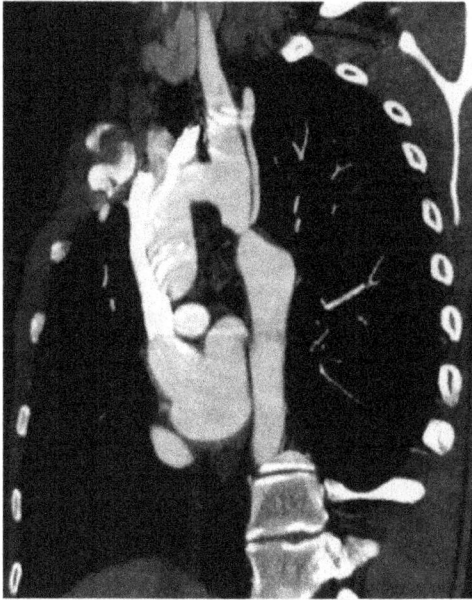

Figure 5. CT angiogram sagittal view of discrete coarctation segment distal to the left subclavian artery.

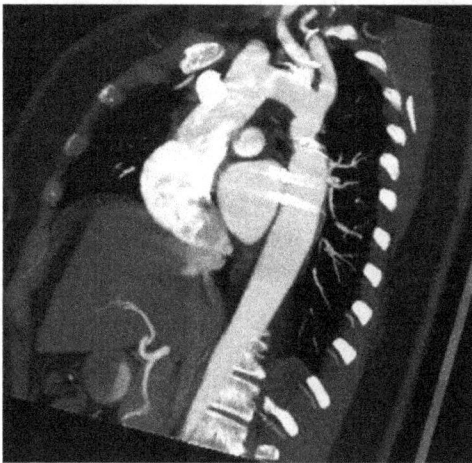

Figure 6. CT angiogram showing recurrent CoA.

aortic arch, follow serial aortic dimensions and can also show associated vascular anomalies such as double superior vena cava or aberrant great vessels. Collateral vessel formation can also be visualized with CTA. The main disadvantage of CTA is radiation exposure, therefore dose-saving algorithms are very important in reducing radiation exposure for patients (**Figures 8–11**).

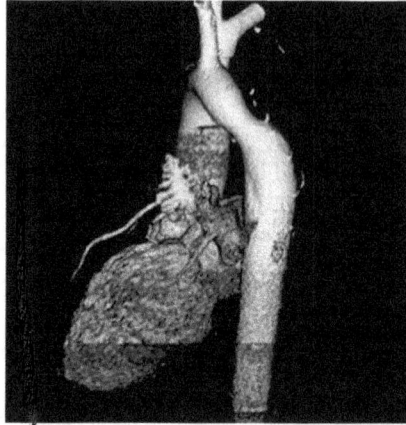

Figure 7. CT 3D reconstruction of the aorta postsurgical repair of CoA.

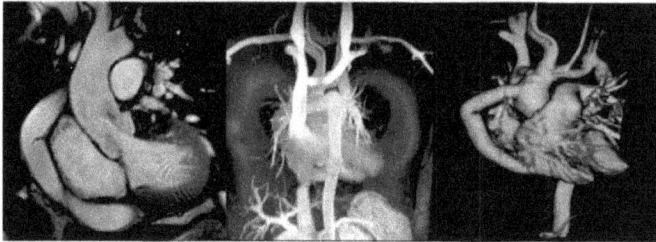

Figure 8. Cardiac MRI of interrupted aortic arch Type A status post a vascular jump graft resulting in a C-shaped appearance of the distal arch and multiple areas of stenosis now with a 20 mm extra-anatomic bypass graft from the mid ascending aorta to the distal descending aorta at the level of the diaphragm. The last picture in this figure shows a three dimensional (3D) reconstructed image of the graft.

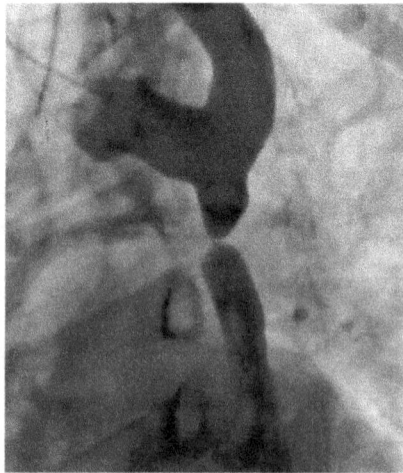

Figure 9. Invasive angiogram showing Type A interruption of the aorta.

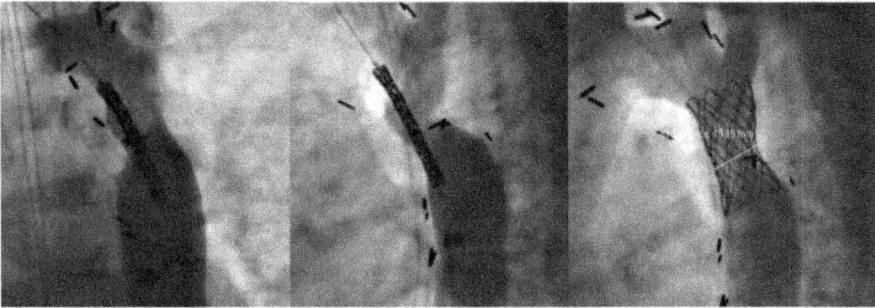

Figure 10. Angiography demonstrating stent placement in a patient with coarctation of the aorta.

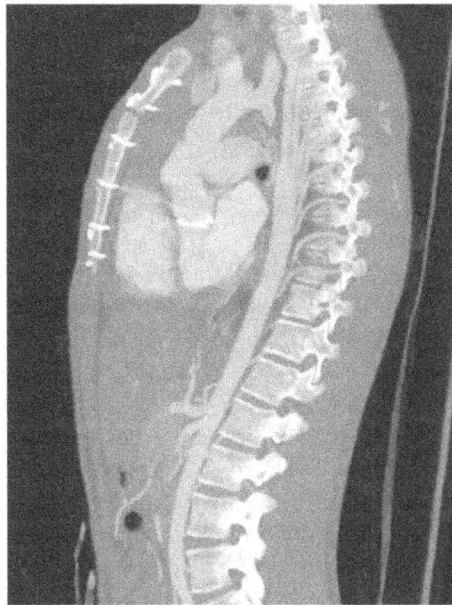

Figure 11. CT angiogram showing Type A interruption of the aortic arch.

9. Management

In 2008, the American College of Cardiology and American Heart Association (ACC/AHA) guidelines for adults with congenital heart disease recommended intervention for coarctation for the following indications:

a. Peak to peak coarctation gradient ≥20 mmHg. The peak to peak gradient is a measurement derived from catheterization data in which the peak pressure beyond the coarctation is subtracted from the peak pressure proximal to the coarctation.

b. Peak to peak coarctation gradient <20 mmHg with anatomic imaging evidence of significant coarctation and radiologic evidence of significant collateral flow [49, 50].

Systemic hypertension, accelerated coronary heart disease, stroke, aortic dissection, and heart failure are common complications in adults who have not undergone correction for their coarctation or were operated on later in life [49]. Coarctation repair after early childhood does not prevent persistence or late recurrence of systemic hypertension. As a result, correction of coarctation should be performed in infancy or early childhood to prevent the development of chronic systemic hypertension [42]. If coarctation escapes early detection, repair should be performed at the time of subsequent diagnosis if clinically indicated. Management with antihypertensive medications is important to prevent long-term complications [2]. According to guidelines, the first line medications in the treatment of hypertension in patients with CoA are angiotensin converting enzyme (ACE) inhibitors, angiotensin-receptor blockers (ARB), and beta blockers (BB) [50]. Hypertension can be treated with medical management, but coarctation or recoarctation of the aorta need to be repaired either percutaneously or surgically [47, 63]. Choosing one intervention over another depends on the individual patient and should be done in collaboration with an interdisciplinary team including an adult congenital heart disease (ACHD) cardiologist, interventionalist and surgeon with training in ACHD. For example, patients with a long segment of coarctation of the aorta, complex arch anatomy, or with interruption of the aorta are more likely to need open-heart surgery as opposed to a transcatheter intervention [64, 65].

9.1. Percutaneous intervention

In the mid-1900s, repair of coarctation of the aorta was entirely surgical. Balloon angioplasty is a percutaneous alternative to surgical repair for older infants and young children (greater than 4 months) with native discrete coarctation. It remains the preferred intervention for all patients with isolated recoarctation regardless of age [49, 66]. However, stent placement has replaced balloon angioplasty as the procedure of choice in older children and adults with native coarctation [66]. Currently, balloon dilatation and stenting remain the transcatheter interventions that can be used for the treatment of CoA [63, 67]. Although balloon angioplasty was the treatment of choice for discrete native coarctation in adults in the past, most centers currently perform stent implantation for older children and adults with native discrete or long-segment coarctation. Through-out the years, continuous advancements in technology and catheter-based techniques have made a variety of percutaneous intervention possibilities available. Improvements in the field have allowed interventions to evolve from balloon angioplasty to endovascular stents to covered stents. The patients who underwent balloon angioplasty were noted to develop residual or recurrent stenosis, aneurysms and dissections or femoral artery complications including occlusion [68]. Stenting, on the other hand, have been shown to be superior to balloon dilatation in relieving the aortic coarctation, with less recurrent narrowing of the aorta, as well as having a smaller amount of complications. Studies have shown that balloon angioplasty and surgical correction are equally effective in reducing the peak systolic pressure gradient early after intervention [69]. The development of covered stents has helped decrease the number of problems associated with injury to the aortic wall and have allowed providers to avoid surgical interventions for aneurysms [2]. Overall, the repair of complex coarctation of the aorta with stents has been shown to be safe with improvements in outcomes [70]. Bare metal stents may be sufficient in many, if not most, patients that undergo stent placement and that further research is needed to determine if there is a subset of patients who truly benefit from the implantation of a covered versus bare stent. Follow-up data will also be important to see if there is a long-term benefit regarding maintaining normal blood pressure using covered stents. Stenting may be less successful in patients with suboptimal anatomy with vessel tortuosity and transverse arch hypoplasia [71]. For these patients, the decision to perform stent placement versus surgical correction must be made on a case-by-case decision by the clinical team.

9.2. Surgical

Resection and direct end-to-end anastomosis or subclavian flap arterioplasty are the most commonly used techniques for the treatment of CoA in the infantile period because anatomic conditions are more favorable. Subclavian flap arterioplasty and patch graft aortoplasty have been developed as an alternative to resection and direct end-to-end anastomosis in which more than one-half of patients experience late-onset re-coarctation problems [72]. However, CoA in adolescents and adults is often complicated with the occurrence of associated comorbidities like aortic aneurysms, dissections, aortic valve disease, and other cardiovascular diseases. Studies actually show that having a BAV is a risk factor for mortality [73]. This is most likely because BAV have been associated with aortic insufficiency and stenosis in addition to dilatation and dissection of the aorta resulting in a potential need for open heart surgery. In a retrospective study of patients with CoA undergoing surgical interventions, aortic aneurysm or dissection and disease of the aortic valve were the most common comorbidities. Within this cohort, 38% had a BAV [72]. Patients with CoA who have left ventricular dysfunction and a brachial-ankle gradient of 20 mmHg or greater have also shown to be at risk for significant cardiovascular events [47]. Earlier, CoA was evaluated as the localization anomaly of the aorta; however, it is currently considered as part of a broad-spectrum pathology. The main goal of surgical treatment in CoA is the removal of stenosis. The surgical technique is selected according to the length of the coarcted segment, localization with the ductus, status of the collateral circulation in the distal aorta, and atherosclerotic alterations in the aortic wall [72]. The resection and graft interposition were first described by Gross in 1951 [74, 75]. This technique is not suitable for pediatric patients, because it restricts the development of the aorta. However, bypass grafting is an appropriate technique particularly for patients with aneurysms, long-segment coarctation or post-recovery aneurysms, and adult patients with diffuse collateral circulation and coarctations. Therefore, artificial bypass grafting was preferred in these patients to prevent complications (i.e., spinal cord complications, bleeding, and aneurysm development) during and after surgery [76]. Prosthetic patch aortoplasty is avoided whenever possible because of the frequent occurrence of aortic aneurysm or rupture [77]. When surgical repair of the coarctation is done at a later age, the possibility of these cardiovascular comorbidities should be kept in mind. Some of the other risks in surgery to consider are related to spinal ischemic injuries and intraoperative bleeding from extensive amounts of collaterals [2]. In general, repair of the CoA surgically has been shown to have a low mortality rate. However, as these patients continue to follow up with their cardiologists, re-coarctation is often seen in the long-term. Other than additional percutaneous procedures, these patients sometimes need to be evaluated for further surgical interventions [78]. Currently, there are no clinical trials showing a direct comparison between transcatheter approaches are superior to surgical interventions or vice versa. More research is needed in this area to compare the different approaches [64].

10. Complications and long-term follow up

All patients with coarctation (repaired or not) should be monitored with lifelong congenital cardiology follow-up and imaging because long-term survival is reduced compared with normative populations and there is potential need for reintervention [79, 80]. The European Society of Cardiology and the American Heart Association recommends continuous life-long follow up of patients with coarctation of the aorta even though they have been repaired [50]. As mentioned previously, even though patients with coarctation are repaired, they are at risk for re-coarctation later in life as well as develop other comorbidities such as hypertension and coronary artery disease. The unoperated mean survival rate of adults with coarctation of the aorta is 35 years of age, with a mortality rate of 75% by 46 years of age [49]. In general, the patients with CoA who are repaired at a later age are more likely to remain hypertensive. This is because in addition to the narrowing of the aorta, they can also develop arterial stiffness and vascular abnormalities asides from alternations in their renin-aldosterone angiotensin system [81]. Investigators have also postulated that the mechanical stress associated with increased pressure load may initiate rapid gene expression for collagen production, leading to re-enforcement and reorganization of the vessel musculo-elastic fascicle, and thereby reducing the degree of pressure-induced aortic dilatation. However, a clear disadvantage of this is that the resultant stiffer vessel will lead to augmented central aortic systolic pressure and systolic hypertension, which is the major cause of longer term morbidity and mortality in these patients, even despite early repair [82].

Other than being hypertensive at rest, it is also common for these patients to be hypertensive with exercise. In a prospective study of 74 patients with coarctation, the systolic blood pressure at peak exercise was an indicator for long term hypertension [83]. Exercise stress testing is useful to assess the patients' hypertensive response, evaluate their need for future interventions and determine prognosis in the long run [84]. Other studies have shown a link between exercise-induced hypertension and left ventricular hypertrophy (LVH) in patients with CoA. LVH has been shown to be associated with a higher incidence of adverse events [85]. Overall, more research is needed in this area to determine the risks and benefits of exercise in patients with CoA and whether there is a need for exercise restrictions. Patients with CoA are also at risk for developing intracranial aneurysms (ICA). With five times the risk of developing ICA, guidelines recommend advanced imaging such as CT or MRI to assess the intracranial vessels. Studies show that screening these patients is reasonable, especially as they get older, since age is one of the main risk factors in the prevalence of ICA [86]. Hypertension will put these patients with aneurysms at risk for cerebrovascular accidents (CVA) and intracranial hemorrhage. In one of the studies comparing patients with congenital heart disease with and without CoA, the patients with CoA (especially adults, men, and the patients without a VSD) have a higher risk of developing hypertension, therefore increasing their risk for CVA [87].

Endocarditis prophylaxis is not required for patients with uncomplicated native coarctation or 6 months after successful repair of native or re-coarctation. Antibiotic prophylaxis is indicated in patients with a past history of endocarditis, in those whose repair involved insertion of a conduit, or for 6 months after intervention if prosthetic material or stent was used. The 2015 scientific statement of the AHA/ACC provides competitive athletic participation guidelines for patients with congenital heart disease (CHD), including coarctation [88]. As with any other guidelines, recommendations need to be tailored to the patient and a comprehensive evaluation by an experienced clinician is required. Before a decision is made regarding sports participation, a detailed evaluation should be conducted, which should include a physical examination, electrocardiography (ECG), chest radiograph, exercise testing, and cardiac/aortic imaging (with transthoracic echocardiogram, MRI, and/or computed tomography angiography [CTA]) when appropriate. The time interval for repeating this extensive testing is unclear and should be individualized to the specific patient.

It is known that morbidity and mortality are higher in patients with CoA given their risk of complications. These patients can have aortic aneurysms, chronic hypertension, re-coarctation, and the potential need for additional transcatheter and surgical interventions. However, for patients with coarctation of the aorta that survive into adulthood, studies have shown that their overall long-term survival rate is high. These patients should be followed up in a center specialized in adult congenital heart disease, where these morbidities are recognized and close observation is provided to prevent devastating complications.

11. Conclusion

Patients with CoA who have undergone repair require lifelong surveillance. Because this type of CHD is associated with many long-term complications, collaborative management by cardiologists with expertise in adult CHD is recommended. As patients with CHD are now surviving into adulthood, with 5–8% of these patients having coarctation of the aorta, it is important to understand the anatomy, pathophysiology, and management of these patients. Although echocardiography is a fundamental tool in the assessment of patients after coarctation repair, advanced imaging is often necessary for comprehensive evaluation. cMRI is the preferred imaging modality for repaired and unrepaired CoA. Alternatively, cardiovascular CT is best suited to evaluate patients with endovascular stents or those with contraindications to cMRI. It is not uncommon for this cohort to develop complications or require additional percutaneous or surgical interventions during their lifetime. This chapter emphasizes the importance of long-term follow up care, especially in a center specializing in the care of patients with congenital heart disease.

Conflict of interest

There is no conflict of interest.

Author details

Ayesha Salahuddin[1,4†], Alice Chan[1,3,4†] and Ali N. Zaidi[1,2,3,4*]

*Address all correspondence to: azaidi@montefiore.org

1 Montefiore Einstein Center for Heart and Vascular Care, Bronx, NY, United States

2 Children's Hospital at Montefiore, Bronx, NY, United States

3 Montefiore Adult Congenital Heart Disease Program (MAtCH), United States

4 Albert Einstein College of Medicine, NY, United States

† These authors contributed equally.

References

[1] Kenny D, Hijazi ZM. Coarctation of the aorta: From fetal life to adulthood. Cardiology Journal. 2011;**18**(5):487-495

[2] Daniels CJ, Zaidi AN. Color Atlas and Synopsis of Adult Congenital Heart Disease. New York: McGraw Hill Education; 2015

[3] Baumgartner H et al. ESC guidelines for the management of grown-up congenital heart disease (new version 2010). European Heart Journal. 2010;**31**(23):2915-2957

[4] Bower C, Ramsay JM. Congenital heart disease: A 10 year cohort. Journal of Paediatrics and Child Health. 1994;**30**(5):414-418

[5] Samanek M, Voriskova M. Congenital heart disease among 815,569 children born between 1980 and 1990 and their 15-year survival: A prospective Bohemia survival study. Pediatric Cardiology. 1999;**20**(6):411-417

[6] Campbell M, Polani PE. The aetiology of coarctation of the aorta. Lancet. 1961;**1**(7175): 463-468

[7] Hoffman JI. Incidence of congenital heart disease: II Prenatal incidence. Pediatric Cardiology. 1995;**16**(4):155-165

[8] Niaz T et al. Incidence, morphology, and progression of bicuspid aortic valve in pediatric and young adult subjects with coexisting congenital heart defects. Congenital Heart Disease. 2017;**12**(3):261-269

[9] Lopez L et al. Turner syndrome is an independent risk factor for aortic dilation in the young. Pediatrics. 2008;**121**(6):e1622-e1627

[10] Rudolph AM, Heymann MA, Spitznas U. Hemodynamic considerations in the development of narrowing of the aorta. The American Journal of Cardiology. 1972;**30**(5):514-525

[11] Ho SY, Anderson RH. Coarctation, tubular hypoplasia, and the ductus arteriosus. Histological study of 35 specimens. British Heart Journal. 1979;**41**(3):268-274

[12] Campbell M. Natural history of coarctation of the aorta. British Heart Journal. 1970;**32**(5): 633-640

[13] Tikkanen J, Heinonen OP. Risk factors for coarctation of the aorta. Teratology. 1993;**47**(6): 565-572

[14] Sehested J. Coarctation of the aorta in monozygotic twins. British Heart Journal. 1982; **47**(6):619-620

[15] Wessels MW et al. Autosomal dominant inheritance of left ventricular outflow tract obstruction. American Journal of Medical Genetics. Part A. 2005;**134A**(2):171-179

[16] Carmeliet P et al. Abnormal blood vessel development and lethality in embryos lacking a single VEGF allele. Nature. 1996;**380**(6573):435-439

[17] Sehested J, Baandrup U, Mikkelsen E. Different reactivity and structure of the prestenotic and poststenotic aorta in human coarctation. Implications for baroreceptor function. Circulation. 1982;**65**(6):1060-1065

[18] McBride KL et al. Inheritance analysis of congenital left ventricular outflow tract obstruction malformations: Segregation, multiplex relative risk, and heritability. American Journal of Medical Genetics. Part A. 2005;**134A**(2):180-186

[19] Cramer JW et al. The spectrum of congenital heart disease and outcomes after surgical repair among children with turner syndrome: A single-center review. Pediatric Cardiology. 2014;**35**(2):253-260

[20] Eckhauser A et al. Turner syndrome in girls presenting with coarctation of the aorta. The Journal of Pediatrics. 2015;**167**(5):1062-1066

[21] Wong SC et al. The prevalence of turner syndrome in girls presenting with coarctation of the aorta. The Journal of Pediatrics. 2014;**164**(2):259-263

[22] Nguyen L, Cook SC. Coarctation of the aorta: Strategies for improving outcomes. Cardiology Clinics. 2015;**33**(4):521-530 vii

[23] Ferencz C et al. Congenital heart disease: Prevalence at livebirth. The Baltimore-Washington infant study. American Journal of Epidemiology. 1985;**121**(1):31-36

[24] McBride KL et al. NOTCH1 mutations in individuals with left ventricular outflow tract malformations reduce ligand-induced signaling. Human Molecular Genetics. 2008;**17**(18):2886-2893

[25] McBride KL et al. Linkage analysis of left ventricular outflow tract malformations (aortic valve stenosis, coarctation of the aorta, and hypoplastic left heart syndrome). European Journal of Human Genetics. 2009;**17**(6):811-819

[26] Pham PP et al. Cardiac catheterization and operative outcomes from a multicenter consortium for children with Williams syndrome. Pediatric Cardiology. 2009;**30**(1):9-14

[27] McBride KL et al. Epidemiology of noncomplex left ventricular outflow tract obstruction malformations (aortic valve stenosis, coarctation of the aorta, hypoplastic left heart syndrome) in Texas, 1999-2001. Birth Defects Research. Part A, Clinical and Molecular Teratology. 2005;**73**(8):555-561

[28] Wren C, Richmond S, Donaldson L. Temporal variability in birth prevalence of cardio-vascular malformations. Heart. 2000;**83**(4):414-419

[29] Reifenstein GH, Levine SA, Gross RE. Coarctation of the aorta; a review of 104 autopsied cases of the adult type, 2 years of age or older. American Heart Journal. 1947;**33**(2):146-168

[30] Mann DL et al. Braunwald's Heart Disease : A Textbook of Cardiovascular Medicine. 10thed ed. Elsevier, Saunders; 2015

[31] Vogt M et al. Impaired elastic properties of the ascending aorta in newborns before and early after successful coarctation repair: Proof of a systemic vascular disease of the pre-stenotic arteries? Circulation. 2005;**111**(24):3269-3273

[32] Becker AE, Becker MJ, Edwards JE. Anomalies associated with coarctation of aorta: Particular reference to infancy. Circulation. 1970;**41**(6):1067-1075

[33] Teo LL et al. Prevalence of associated cardiovascular abnormalities in 500 patients with aortic coarctation referred for cardiovascular magnetic resonance imaging to a tertiary center. Pediatric Cardiology. 2011;**32**(8):1120-1127

[34] Johnson D et al. Resetting of the cardiopulmonary baroreflex 10 years after surgical repair of coarctation of the aorta. Heart. 2001;**85**(3):318-325

[35] de Divitiis M, Rubba P, Calabro R. Arterial hypertension and cardiovascular prognosis after successful repair of aortic coarctation: A clinical model for the study of vascular function. Nutrition, Metabolism, and Cardiovascular Diseases. 2005;**15**(5):382-394

[36] de Divitiis M et al. Vascular dysfunction after repair of coarctation of the aorta: Impact of early surgery. Circulation. 2001;**104**(12 Suppl 1):I165-I1170

[37] Pedersen TA et al. High pulse pressure is not associated with abnormal activation of the renin-angiotensin-aldosterone system in repaired aortic coarctation. Journal of Human Hypertension. 2015;**29**(4):268-273

[38] Martinez-Maldonado M et al. Aortic and renal regulation of the renin-angiotensin system in interrenal aortic coarctation. Transactions of the Association of American Physicians. 1993;**106**:120-127

[39] Kenny D et al. Hypertension and coarctation of the aorta: An inevitable consequence of developmental pathophysiology. Hypertension Research. 2011;**34**(5):543-547

[40] Cohen M et al. Coarctation of the aorta. Long-term follow-up and prediction of outcome after surgical correction. Circulation. 1989;**80**(4):840-545

[41] Clarkson PM et al. Results after repair of coarctation of the aorta beyond infancy: A 10 to 28 year follow-up with particular reference to late systemic hypertension. The American Journal of Cardiology. 1983;**51**(9):1481-1488

[42] Seirafi PA et al. Repair of coarctation of the aorta during infancy minimizes the risk of late hypertension. The Annals of Thoracic Surgery. 1998;**66**(4):1378-1382

[43] Tobian L Jr. A viewpoint concerning the enigma of hypertension. The American Journal of Medicine. 1972;**52**(5):595-609

[44] O'Sullivan JJ, Derrick G, Darnell R. Prevalence of hypertension in children after early repair of coarctation of the aorta: A cohort study using casual and 24 hour blood pressure measurement. Heart. 2002;**88**(2):163-166

[45] Canniffe C et al. Hypertension after repair of aortic coarctation—A systematic review. International Journal of Cardiology. 2013;**167**(6):2456-2461

[46] Bald M, Neudorf U. Arterial hypertension in children and adolescents after surgical repair of aortic coarctation defined by ambulatory blood pressure monitoring. Blood Pressure Monitoring. 2000;**5**(3):163-167

[47] Bambul Heck P et al. Survival and cardiovascular events after coarctation-repair in long-term follow-up (COAFU): Predictive value of clinical variables. International Journal of Cardiology. 2017;**228**:347-351

[48] Jenkins NP, Ward C. Coarctation of the aorta: Natural history and outcome after surgical treatment. QJM. 1999;**92**(7):365-371

[49] Warnes CA et al. ACC/AHA 2008 guidelines for the Management of adults with congenital heart disease: A report of the American College of Cardiology/American Heart Association task force on practice guidelines (writing committee to develop guidelines on the management of adults with congenital heart disease). Circulation. 2008;**118**(23):e714-e833

[50] Warnes CA et al. ACC/AHA 2008 guidelines for the management of adults with congenital heart disease: Executive summary: A report of the American College of Cardiology/American Heart Association task force on practice guidelines (writing committee to develop guidelines for the management of adults with congenital heart disease). Circulation. 2008;**118**(23):2395-2451

[51] Krieger EV et al. Comparison of risk of hypertensive complications of pregnancy among women with versus without coarctation of the aorta. The American Journal of Cardiology. 2011;**107**(10):1529-1534

[52] Vriend JW et al. Outcome of pregnancy in patients after repair of aortic coarctation. European Heart Journal. 2005;**26**(20):2173-2178

[53] Beauchesne LM et al. Coarctation of the aorta: Outcome of pregnancy. Journal of the American College of Cardiology. 2001;**38**(6):1728-1733

[54] Engvall J et al. Arm-ankle systolic blood pressure difference at rest and after exercise in the assessment of aortic coarctation. British Heart Journal. 1995;**73**(3):270-276

[55] Marx GR, Allen HD. Accuracy and pitfalls of Doppler evaluation of the pressure gradient in aortic coarctation. Journal of the American College of Cardiology. 1986;**7**(6):1379-1385

[56] Jae K, Oh JBS, Jamil Tajik A. Echo Manual. 3rd ed. Philadelphia: Lippincott Williams &Wilkins; 2007

[57] Houston AB et al. Doppler ultrasound in the assessment of severity of coarctation of the aorta and interruption of the aortic arch. British Heart Journal. 1987;**57**(1):38-43

[58] Silvilairat S et al. Abdominal aortic pulsed wave Doppler patterns reliably reflect clinical severity in patients with coarctation of the aorta. Congenital Heart Disease. 2008;**3**(6):422-430

[59] Nielsen JC et al. Magnetic resonance imaging predictors of coarctation severity. Circulation. 2005;**111**(5):622-628

[60] Shepherd B et al. MRI in adult patients with aortic coarctation: Diagnosis and follow-up. Clinical Radiology. 2015;**70**(4):433-445

[61] Goldberg A, Jha S. Phase-contrast MRI and applications in congenital heart disease. Clinical Radiology. 2012;**67**(5):399-410

[62] Hope MD et al. Clinical evaluation of aortic coarctation with 4D flow MR imaging. Journal of Magnetic Resonance Imaging. 2010;**31**(3):711-718

[63] Salcher M et al. Balloon dilatation and stenting for aortic coarctation: A systematic review and meta-analysis. Circulation. Cardiovascular Interventions. 2016;**9**(6)

[64] Padua LM et al. Stent placement versus surgery for coarctation of the thoracic aorta. Cochrane Database of Systematic Reviews. 2012;**5**:CD008204

[65] Forbes TJ et al. Comparison of surgical, stent, and balloon angioplasty treatment of native coarctation of the aorta: An observational study by the CCISC (congenital cardiovascular interventional study consortium). Journal of the American College of Cardiology. 2011;**58**(25):2664-2674

[66] Feltes TF et al. Indications for cardiac catheterization and intervention in pediatric cardiac disease: A scientific statement from the American Heart Association. Circulation. 2011;**123**(22):2607-2652

[67] Zussman ME et al. Transcatheter intervention for coarctation of the aorta. Cardiology in the Young. 2016;**26**(8):1563-1567

[68] Fawzy ME et al. Twenty-two years of follow-up results of balloon angioplasty for discreet native coarctation of the aorta in adolescents and adults. American Heart Journal. 2008;**156**(5):910-917

[69] Cowley CG et al. Long-term, randomized comparison of balloon angioplasty and surgery for native coarctation of the aorta in childhood. Circulation. 2005;**111**(25):3453-3456

[70] Suarez de Lezo J et al. Stent repair for complex coarctation of aorta. JACC. Cardiovascular Interventions. 2015;**8**(10):1368-1379

[71] Silversides CK et al. Canadian cardiovascular society 2009 consensus conference on the management of adults with congenital heart disease: Outflow tract obstruction, coarctation of the aorta, tetralogy of Fallot, Ebstein anomaly and Marfan's syndrome. The Canadian Journal of Cardiology. 2010;**26**(3):e80-e97

[72] Yin K et al. Surgical management of aortic coarctation in adolescents and adults. Interactive Cardiovascular and Thoracic Surgery. 2017;**24**(3):430-435

[73] Ozbaydar M et al. Arthroscopic reconstruction of the rotator cuff. The current gold standard? Orthopade. 2007;**36**(9):825-833

[74] van Son JA, Daniels O, Lacquet LK. Current viewpoints concerning the surgical treatment of aortic coarctation in infants and children. Nederlands Tijdschrift voor Geneeskunde. 1990;**134**(35):1682-1688

[75] van Heurn LW et al. Surgical treatment of aortic coarctation in infants younger than three months: 1985 to 1990. Success of extended end-to-end arch aortoplasty. The Journal of Thoracic and Cardiovascular Surgery. 1994;**107**(1):74-85 discussion 85-6

[76] Kaya U et al. Surgical management of aortic coarctation from infant to adult. The Eurasian journal of medicine. 2018;**50**(1):14-18

[77] Parks WJ et al. Incidence of aneurysm formation after Dacron patch aortoplasty repair for coarctation of the aorta: Long-term results and assessment utilizing magnetic resonance angiography with three-dimensional surface rendering. Journal of the American College of Cardiology. 1995;**26**(1):266-271

[78] Noly PE et al. Results of a multimodal approach for the management of aortic coarctation and its complications in adults. Interactive Cardiovascular and Thoracic Surgery. 2017;**25**(3):335-342

[79] Brown ML et al. Coarctation of the aorta: Lifelong surveillance is mandatory following surgical repair. Journal of the American College of Cardiology. 2013;**62**(11):1020-1025

[80] Manganas C et al. Reoperation and coarctation of the aorta: The need for lifelong surveillance. The Annals of Thoracic Surgery. 2001;**72**(4):1222-1224

[81] Morgan GJ et al. Systemic blood pressure after stent management for arch coarctation implications for clinical care. JACC. Cardiovascular Interventions. 2013;**6**(2):192-201

[82] Laurent S et al. Expert consensus document on arterial stiffness: Methodological issues and clinical applications. European Heart Journal. 2006;**27**(21):2588-2605

[83] Luijendijk P et al. Usefulness of exercise-induced hypertension as predictor of chronic hypertension in adults after operative therapy for aortic isthmic coarctation in childhood. The American Journal of Cardiology. 2011;**108**(3):435-439

[84] Foulds HJA et al. A systematic review and meta-analysis of exercise and exercise hypertension in patients with aortic coarctation. Journal of Human Hypertension. 2017;**31**(12):768-775

[85] Krieger EV et al. Correlation of exercise response in repaired coarctation of the aorta to left ventricular mass and geometry. The American Journal of Cardiology. 2013;**111**(3):406-411

[86] Cook SC et al. Assessment of the cerebral circulation in adults with coarctation of the aorta. Congenital Heart Disease. 2013;**8**(4):289-295

[87] Wu MH et al. Risk of systemic hypertension and cerebrovascular accident in patients with aortic Coarctation aged <60 years (from a National Database Study). The American Journal of Cardiology. 2015;**116**(5):779-784

[88] Van Hare GF et al. Eligibility and disqualification recommendations for competitive athletes with cardiovascular abnormalities: Task force 4: Congenital heart disease: A scientific statement from the American Heart Association and American College of Cardiology. Journal of the American College of Cardiology. 2015;**66**(21):2372-2384

www.ingramcontent.com/pod-product-compliance
Lightning Source LLC
Chambersburg PA
CBHW081236190326
41458CB00016B/5798